SMART
PUMPING

for people with diabetes

Editor

Howard A. Wolpert, MD

Contributors

Barbara J. Anderson, PhD is a psychologist and researcher whose work has focused on interventions in the health care system to support personal and family adaptation to diabetes. She is currently Associate Professor in Pediatrics at Baylor College of Medicine in Houston, and co-editor of Practical Psychology for Diabetes Clinicians published by the ADA.

Karen Hanson Chalmers, MS, RD, CDE is the Director of Nutrition Services and the Coordinator of the Insulin Pump Program at the Joslin Diabetes Center in Boston. She is a Board Member of the National Certification Board of Diabetes Educators, and is co-author of the ADA published 16 Myths of a "Diabetic Diet."

Maria C. Gallego, MEd, RD, CDE is a dietitian and diabetes educator who specializes in insulin pump therapy. She is currently Manager of Clinical Services for the Animas Corporation in eastern New England, and prior to this was the Coordinator of the Insulin Pump Program at the Joslin Diabetes Center in Boston. Maria has had diabetes for 12 years, and has used an insulin pump for 6 years.

Cathy A. Mullooly, MS, RCEP, CDE is the Director of Exercise Physiology at the Joslin Diabetes Center in Boston. Cathy currently represents the field of exercise physiology in several diabetes-related capacities, including the National Board of Diabetes Educators and the ADA Program Publication Editorial Board.

Howard A. Wolpert, MD is Senior Physician in the Section of Adult Diabetes and Director of the Insulin Pump Program at the Joslin Diabetes Center in Boston. He is currently collaborating with Dr. Barbara Anderson on a forthcoming ADA guide book about working with young adults who have diabetes.

SMART PUMPING

for people with diabetes

Howard Wolpert, MD, Editor

American Diabetes Association.

Cure • Care • Commitment™

Director, Book Publishing, John Fedor; *Associate Director, Consumer Books,* Sherrye Landrum; *Editor,* Abe Ogden; *Production Manager,* Peggy M. Rote; *Composition,* Circle Graphics, Inc.; *Cover Design,* Koncept, Inc; *Printer,* Port City Press, Inc.

Printed in the United States of America

3 5 7 9 10 8 6 4

The suggestions and information contained in this publication are generally consistent with the *Clinical Practice Recommendations* and other policies of the American Diabetes Association, but they do not represent the policy or position of the Association or any of its boards or committees. Reasonable steps have been taken to ensure the accuracy of the information presented. However, the American Diabetes Association cannot ensure the safety or efficacy of any product or service described in this publication. Individuals are advised to consult a physician or other appropriate health care professional before undertaking any diet or exercise program or taking any medication referred to in this publication. Professionals must use and apply their own professional judgment, experience, and training and should not rely solely on the information contained in this publication before prescribing any diet, exercise, or medication. The American Diabetes Association—its officers, directors, employees, volunteers, and members—assumes no responsibility or liability for personal or other injury, loss, or damage that may result from the suggestions or information in this publication.

⊚ The paper in this publication meets the requirements of the ANSI Standard Z39.48-1992 (permanence of paper).

ADA titles may be purchased for business or promotional use or for special sales. To purchase this book in large quantities, or for custom editions of this book with your logo, contact Lee Romano Sequeira, Special Sales & Promotions, at the address below, or at LRomano@diabetes.org or 703-299-2046.

American Diabetes Association
1701 North Beauregard Street
Alexandria, Virginia 22311

Library of Congress Cataloging-in-Publication Data

Smart pumping : a practical approach to mastering the insulin pump / editor, Howard A. Wolpert.
    p. cm.
  Includes index.
  ISBN 1-58040-125-2 (pbk. : alk. paper)
    1. Insulin pumps—Popular works. I. Wolpert, Howard A., 1958-

RC 661.I63 S63 2002
616.4'62061—dc21

                                          2002026211

Dedication

This book is dedicated to Karl B. Smith, Jr., a man whose vitality and courage gives us a vision of diabetes that inspires confidence and hope. The young Karl Smith was diagnosed with diabetes at age 6 in 1922— the year Dr. Frederick Banting and his associates first isolated insulin. Mr. Smith's life with diabetes has been an example of what the Diabetes Control and Complications Trial later proved. Decades ago at his own initiative, he changed to a multiple daily insulin injection regimen to regulate his diabetes.

But as we all know, success in living with diabetes is about more than glucose levels and A1C measurements. It's about a spirit of courage and resilience, dauntless drive, and refusing to allow diabetes to be a barrier to the fullest pursuit and celebration of life. That is the example of Karl Smith—in his 79th year with diabetes he is still playing paddle tennis. He has set a trail we expect others will follow.

Contents

Acknowledgments

This book grew out of educational materials used in the Pump Program at the Joslin Diabetes Center. Special thanks go to the hundreds of patients whose experiences, observations, and questions helped shape the perspectives and insights presented in this book and to Abe Ogden and Sherrye Landrum for their important editorial guidance.

Introduction

Finding balance between the demands of managing diabetes and enjoying the pleasures of life is the challenge faced by every person with diabetes. In this book, *Smart Pumping: A Practical Approach to Mastering the Insulin Pump*, we present a "post-post-DCCT perspective" on what insulin pumps and the tools of intensive diabetes management offer to people with diabetes. What do we mean by this? The Diabetes Control and Complications Trial (DCCT) was a landmark study that established that good glucose control can reduce the risk for long-term complications from diabetes. In the immediate "post-DCCT era," the message has been that *metabolic control matters*. However, many patients have told us that this focus on blood glucose control can make it seem as if the quality of their life is only of secondary importance and ignores the major challenge faced in their daily life—making diabetes manageable. Intensive diabetes management does require extra effort and sometimes inconvenience, but quality of life doesn't need to be sacrificed in order to achieve good metabolic control. The "post-post-DCCT perspective" presented in this book views pumps not simply as a means to improve glucose control, but also as tools that can make diabetes more manageable and can offer you immediate lifestyle benefits and freedom.

We have structured this book into three parts and tried to create a guide that corresponds with the journey most people take with the insulin pump:

- **Section I:** *Why Bother with the Pump?*, which presents our perspective on what the tools of intensive diabetes management offer you and the pros and cons of pumping.
- **Section II:** *Mastering Pump Basics*, which outlines a road map for getting started on the pump and the essential skills for safe and effective pumping. This section may also be of interest to those already pumping who want to review the fundamentals.
- **Section III:** *Beyond the Basics: Intensive Management and Pump Use in the Real World* touches on a range of issues. Some of the chapters may be of value to all people on the pump (Chapter 10:

"Understanding Insulin: How It Acts and How You Respond"), while other chapters may be only of interest to some (Chapter 12: "Intensive Therapy, Weight Gain, and Getting More Out of Your Exercise").

Today, insulin pumps are technically more advanced, smaller, and more versatile. Yet current pumps are not "smarter" than the pumps of the 1980s and 1990s. Rather, current pumps are tools that continue to depend on the "smarts" of the pump user and his or her health care providers. *Smart Pumping* isn't intended to be only a technical manual of pump do's and don'ts. In this book, we emphasize that being "smart" about pump therapy includes: technical skills in diabetes self-management, an appreciation that pump use is *not* a "quick fix" to get on track, and an acceptance that frustrations and lapses are an inevitable part of everyone's life journey with diabetes and *not* a sign of personal failure.

The challenges of managing diabetes from day to day are inseparable from the complexities of life. In this book, we have set out to cover both the technical and behavioral aspects of pump therapy and to present an integrated perspective. We hope that you will hear one voice—the voice of a diabetes coach, a hybrid physician/psychologist/pump trainer/nutritionist/exercise physiologist—who believes that success in mastering the insulin pump depends on technical skills, practice, realistic goals, positive reinforcement, and knowing how to pace yourself.

I

Why Bother with the Pump?

1

You Don't Need a Sermon

But the Basics Don't Hurt

There's a good chance that from the very minute you were diagnosed with diabetes, you've been overwhelmed with information. Information that's been pretty much telling you the same thing—get your blood sugars under control and your chances for a long and complication-free life dramatically increase. We could give examples, such as the Diabetes Control and Complications Trial (DCCT), where over 1,400 individuals with diabetes were divided into 2 groups: a "conventional" group that took up to 2 insulin injections a day and an "intensive" group that used multiple insulin injections or an insulin pump. As you've probably already guessed, the intensive group ended up in a lot better shape. In fact, they had less than half as many severe eye, kidney, and nerve complications as those in the conventional group (Fig. 1-1).

But you probably already knew this. Maybe not specifically, but you had a good idea that good blood glucose control means healthier living. So you don't need any more sermons from health professionals. You know *why* you need good glucose control. That's not the hard part. The challenge is how you achieve good control and how you balance the day-to-day demands of diabetes with the other demands (and pleasures!) of life.

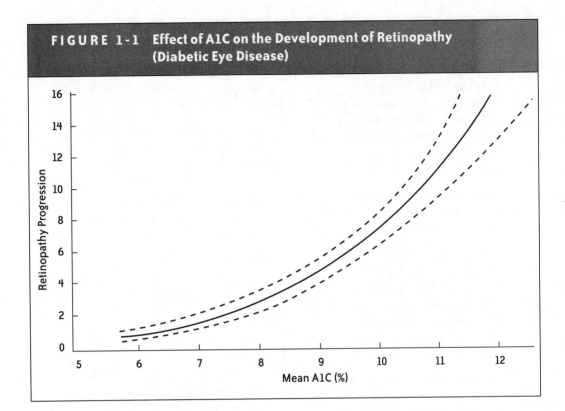

FIGURE 1-1   **Effect of A1C on the Development of Retinopathy (Diabetic Eye Disease)**

Understanding the Challenge in Achieving Good Control

Before we start talking about how to achieve good blood sugar control, it's probably best if we cover the basics about how insulin regulates glucose metabolism in the body. The more you understand the mechanics of diabetes, the better prepared you are to take control.

As you probably know, insulin is a hormone that most people naturally produce in the pancreas (Fig. 1-2).

Basically, there are 2 sides to the insulin coin:

- Background insulin (also known in pump therapy as *basal insulin*, which we'll soon cover) controls the blood glucose levels between meals and overnight. During these periods, the liver (which acts like the body's glucose "reservoir") is continuously releasing glucose into the bloodstream to provide energy for basic functions in your body. Insulin helps control this process. Without basal insulin, your liver would release glucose into the

Some Facts about the A1C

▌ The A1C (pronounced "ay-one-see") gives you a weighted mean for your blood glucose levels over the past 3 months. This test actually measures the amount of glucose that attaches to hemoglobin, which is a protein in the red blood cells.

▌ Every 1% drop in A1C is associated with about a 40% reduction in risk for diabetic eye disease (retinopathy).

▌ People without diabetes have A1C levels below 6.0%. The A1C level in the person with diabetes is an important measure of how well the glucose levels are controlled. Very few individuals with diabetes manage to keep the A1C in the "normal" nondiabetic range.

▌ The trade-off for keeping your A1C too low can be an increased likelihood for low blood sugar (hypoglycemic) reactions.

▌ Achieving tight glucose control isn't easy: the average A1C for patients in the "intensive" group of the DCCT was between 7.0 and 7.2%, and for the adolescents in the "intensive" group, it was 8.1%.

▌ To calculate your glucose level for the past 3 months from your A1C, simply multiply your A1C by 22.

For example, an A1C of 7.0% is equal to an average glucose level of 154 mg/dl (7.0 × 22 = 154).

(If you live in a country where glucose is measured in mmol/l rather than mg/dl, multiply your A1C by 1.2 to get your glucose level in mmol/l. All blood glucose measurements in this book are in mg/dl; to convert to mmol/l, divide by 18.)

▌ To bring your A1C down by 1% you would need to lower your average glucose level by 22 mg/dl.

For example, to bring your A1C down from 8.5% to 7.5%, you would only need to lower your average glucose from 187 mg/dl (8.5 × 22) to 165 mg/dl (7.5 × 22).

That's not that big of a change. Good diabetes control really is in your reach!

▌ Putting all of this information together may help you realize that even modest improvements in your glucose control can have a major impact on your future health. Reducing your A1C by 0.5% (the same as lowering your average glucose reading by only 11 mg/dl) will lower your risk for eye disease from diabetes by 20%!

bloodstream, but your cells wouldn't be able to get to it. As a result, your blood glucose level would rise rapidly. In addition, your liver would start producing ketone bodies that would build up in the bloodstream, sending you into *diabetic ketoacidosis*. This is a very dangerous condition.

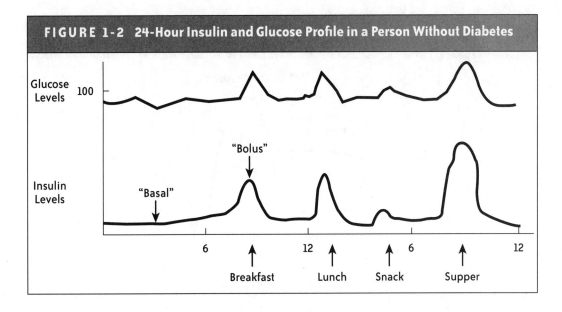

FIGURE 1-2   24-Hour Insulin and Glucose Profile in a Person Without Diabetes

■ Insulin surges at mealtimes when blood sugar rises (known in pump therapy as *boluses*) cause the tissues of the body to take up glucose from the bloodstream. The amount of insulin produced in these mealtime surges are very precisely controlled to make sure that there is just enough to take care of the carbohydrates being eaten. Eat a bit more, and more insulin is produced; eat a bit less, and less insulin is produced.

So What if Your Body Doesn't Effectively Produce Insulin?

Insulin treatment—the old way

The old (and unfortunately still common) approach to insulin treatment is very rigid. To keep your glucose levels under good control, you're required to organize your life, routine, and eating patterns around your insulin profiles. The following list of activities may sound woefully familiar:

■ Lunch has to be eaten at a specific time, or else the insulin kicks in, along with hypoglycemia.
■ Snacks have to be eaten between meals to keep the long-acting insulin from causing hypoglycemia.

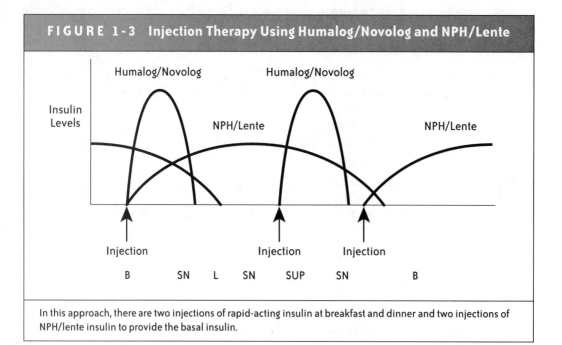

FIGURE 1-3   Injection Therapy Using Humalog/Novolog and NPH/Lente

In this approach, there are two injections of rapid-acting insulin at breakfast and dinner and two injections of NPH/lente insulin to provide the basal insulin.

■ Meals and snacks must have consistent carbohydrate (carb) content, or else your insulin can't handle the carbohydrate load and blood sugars rise.

■ You have to get up at the same time every morning because the longer-acting insulin you took at bedtime is starting to run thin. Sleeping-in means high blood sugars.

Sounds great doesn't it! Having a leisurely weekend or laid-back vacation day to do whatever suits your fancy just doesn't fit in with this old insulin regimen. There's no chance for brunch or getting up late, and Thanksgiving dinners are a problem.

With this method of insulin therapy, good glucose control means you are forced to let diabetes control your life, and that's a pretty rough trade-off.

Insulin therapy—the new way

Thankfully, self-monitoring of blood glucose, the development of insulin pumps, and newer insulins have started to change this rigid therapy structure. In fact, new methods have brought us closer to actually mimicking the way the pancreas produces and releases insulin in the body (Fig. 1-4).

With all of these new tools, insulin therapy has become much more liberating. Following are just a few of the advantages of more progressive insulin therapy:

- You can match the amount of insulin you take to the amount of food you eat, and you can eat whenever you want. Plus, you don't need snacks between meals to stave off hypoglycemia.
- Using the pump, you can drop your background insulin levels when you exercise. This makes burning calories a lot easier.
- You can sleep in late!

Obviously, things are looking brighter. New approaches are giving people with diabetes more and more flexibility. Instead of having to live your life around your insulin regimen, you can design an insulin regimen that fits in with the life you want to live.

So how does the pump fit in with all of this?

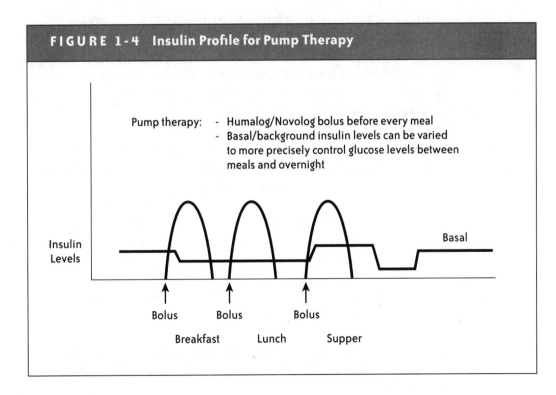

FIGURE 1-4   Insulin Profile for Pump Therapy

Pump therapy: - Humalog/Novolog bolus before every meal
- Basal/background insulin levels can be varied to more precisely control glucose levels between meals and overnight

Insulin Levels

Basal

Bolus   Bolus   Bolus

Breakfast   Lunch   Supper

2 The Pump Advantage

As we talked about in the last chapter, a variety of improvements in insulin therapy have led to more flexibility and freedom for people who need insulin. As a result, both multiple insulin injections and insulin pumps help you build a regimen that's right for you. So why bother with the expense and learning curve of the pump if you can just start using better insulin? Well, there are lots of reasons.

- Pumps deliver insulin much more precisely than injections, which can be especially helpful if you only take very small amounts of insulin at a time.
- Pumps eliminate the need for longer-acting insulins, which are generally absorbed unpredictably in your body.
- Pumps also allow you to vary the amount of background insulin you have in your bloodstream. This leads to much more stable glucose levels between meals and overnight. Naturally, this is better for anyone who uses insulin, but is especially helpful if you:

  - Have high blood glucose in the morning, even if your glucose is right on target when you go to bed. This is often related to the *dawn phenomenon*, a period in the early morning when your liver releases increased amounts of glucose into the bloodstream.

- Have frequent low blood sugar reactions, particularly if your ability to detect hypoglycemia has been dulled (*hypoglycemia unawareness*. See below).
- Have gastroparesis and tend to eat erratically when your symptoms flare up (See below).
- Have difficulty controlling your glucose levels during physical activity.

■ If you eat out a lot, pumps can be a lifesaver. Generally, restaurant food is higher in fat and this can cause your glucose to sky-rocket. Even worse, there's no guarantee on when your food will actually get to you. With a pump, you can spread out your meal-time insulin (we'll talk about how later on) and/or use a *temporary* basal (see page 23) to match your insulin to the amount and type of food you're eating.

■ Losing weight can be much easier when you're on the pump. Since you don't have to eat predetermined amounts of food at predetermined times, changing your eating patterns to accommodate for healthy fare is easier. You can also drop your basal insulin level during exercise, which means you don't have to snack as much and can use exercise to burn off calories and lose weight.

■ If your insulin sensitivity fluctuates at different times in your menstrual cycle, a pump may make it much easier to regulate your glucose levels.

■ The pump can be a lot less hassle. Instead of taking 4 or more injections every day, you change a catheter site every 2–3 days. Which would you prefer?

Insulin Glargine (Lantus) vs. the Pump

In 2001, a virtually peakless, long-acting insulin glargine was introduced that offered much more stable insulin and glucose levels than its long-acting predecessors. With the instability of long-acting insulin apparently improved, many people with diabetes began to wonder what advantages the pump now had over multiple insulin injections. Basically, it has many of the advantages already mentioned above. This new insulin glargine made for better insulin absorption over a long period of time, but still didn't help with fluctuating insulin sensitivity (in particular, the *dawn phenomenon*), the challenges of restaurant eating, and problems posed by exercise. Insulin glargine significantly improves intensive insulin therapy, but there's a good chance you're going to get better over-all control with the pump. Lastly, insulin glargine still requires you to take at least 4 injections every day for good control. Glargine is used to cover basal insulin requirements, and injections of short-acting insulin are needed to cover meals and snacks and to "correct" high blood glucose levels.

The Downside to the Pump: Ketoacidosis, Catheter-Site Infections, and the Expense

Clearly, there are many reasons why people choose pump therapy to achieve flexibility and good diabetes control. However, there are down-sides to using the pump—the most significant of which is a higher risk for ketoacidosis. In addition, infections can sometimes develop where the pump catheter passes through your skin.

As discussed in Chapter 1, insulin has a key role in controlling your liver from producing ketones. When insulin levels in the bloodstream drop, your liver is triggered to start producing ketone bodies. This sit-uation can rapidly develop into a condition called *ketoacidosis*. With pump therapy, long-acting insulin is not used, and so any accidental interruption of delivery of short-acting insulin from your pump can result in ketoacidosis. This is a potential problem only if you have type 1 diabetes. If you have type 2 diabetes and your pancreas is still producing some insulin, you are unlikely to develop ketoacidosis if insulin delivery by the pump stops. For tips on how to detect and prevent ketoacidosis, see Chapter 9.

The skin is a natural barrier against infection. The catheter through which the pump delivers insulin passes through the skin, and this can become a route for bacteria to cause skin infections. This is rare and typically occurs if the catheter is left in place for too long and if your glucose levels are running high. For tips on how to reduce your risk for skin infections and how to recognize and treat these infections, see Chapter 7.

Pump therapy is expensive: The average price for the pump is around $5,000, and then there's an additional $1,500+ per year for dis-posables, such as the infusion sets, reservoirs (syringes), and batteries. Some states have laws mandating that insurance companies cover these expenses. Check with your insurance company or the pump company to find out how much of these expenses will be covered.

Added Bonuses: The Pump and Hypoglycemia Unawareness

As you may already be aware, one of the more dangerous side effects of striving for lower average glucose levels is an increased occurrence of low blood sugar reactions, or hypoglycemia. We all know the dangers and symptoms of hypoglycemia, most of which can impair your ability to safely conduct common activities, such as driving a car. What you may not be aware of, however, are the more subtle problems that can arise from frequent hypoglycemia. Behavioral changes, for instance, are a common result of this condition. Irritation, anger, and irrationality are just a few side effects. One more dangerous side effect is the inability to detect hypoglycemia entirely, a condition known as *hypoglycemia unawareness*.

What is hypoglycemia unawareness?

Basically, hypoglycemia unawareness is a condition that dulls your body's reaction to low blood sugar attacks. You become unaware of the hypoglycemia. The most dangerous and alarming aspect of hypo-glycemia unawareness is that the cause is also the effect and a vicious cycle is created. Frequent hypoglycemia causes unawareness, which in turn leads to frequent hypoglycemia.

Surprisingly, it doesn't take long for this cycle to get started. Studies have shown that after a single episode of hypoglycemia, warning signs in your body are muted if another reaction occurs the next day. In other words, it only takes one episode to get the chain reaction started. Before long, you could be looking at a situation something like that in Fig. 2-1.

How the pump can help

This cycle can be stopped. Studies have shown that even though just one hypoglycemic reaction can start dulling warning signs, reducing the frequency of these reactions can help you get these warning signs back. Hypoglycemia unawareness can be reversed. Getting your blood sugars under control can dramatically improve this condition.

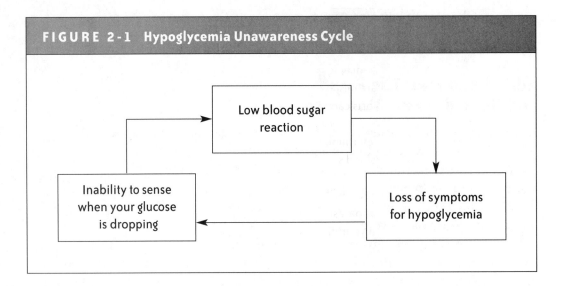

FIGURE 2-1   Hypoglycemia Unawareness Cycle

This is where the pump comes in. Pump therapy means no more long-acting insulin, which in turn means that your insulin and glucose levels tend to be much more stable and predictable. This extra control can give you tight glucose management with less likelihood of accidental hypoglycemia. Pretty soon, not only will you be able to have fewer low blood sugar reactions, but you'll more easily notice when your sugar is too low.

Caution!

If you have hypoglycemia unawareness and are starting pump therapy, make sure your initial basal settings are low and your blood glucose targets are a bit higher than normal. While this may mean higher than normal blood sugars at first, it protects against unnoticed low blood sugar reactions.

Pump Therapy and Gastroparesis

Pump therapy can also help with one of the more unpleasant complications of diabetes—*diabetic gastroparesis*, sometimes referred to as neuropathy of the stomach. Occasionally, people with diabetes have trouble digesting what they eat, and the food ends up sitting in their stomach for

Don't Jump to Conclusions

Gastroparesis is often over-diagnosed, meaning that a lot of people who don't have gastroparesis are mistakenly told they have the condition. High blood sugar and ketoacidosis can also cause a delayed emptying of your stomach and produce the same symptoms. Furthermore, if the gastric emptying test doctors use to determine whether or not you have gastroparesis is performed while your blood sugar is high, the results could mistakenly point to gastroparesis.

So just because you have the symptoms doesn't necessarily mean you're suffering from gastroparesis. Your glucose control just may not be as tight as it should. Talk with your diabetes care team to be certain.

too long. This is gastroparesis, and it results from damage to the nerve cells that control the emptying of your stomach. Symptoms include:

- Nausea
- Vomiting
- Poor appetite
- Feeling bloated or full after eating only a very small amount
- Having low blood glucose levels after eating when you've taken insulin

As you can imagine, having food sit in your stomach after you eat can create some serious problems with your insulin therapy. One of the keys to good glucose control is making sure your insulin bolus peaks at the same time as most of the glucose from your meal is being absorbed. If your stomach isn't emptying properly, the glucose from your meal is going to be absorbed unpredictably. How can you match your insulin with something you can't predict? You can't, and your blood glucose control is going to slip.

Suddenly, you find yourself in another vicious cycle. Instead of low blood sugars leading to more low blood sugars, you get high blood sugars leading to more high blood sugars (Fig. 2-2). It's the same principle, just the other way around.

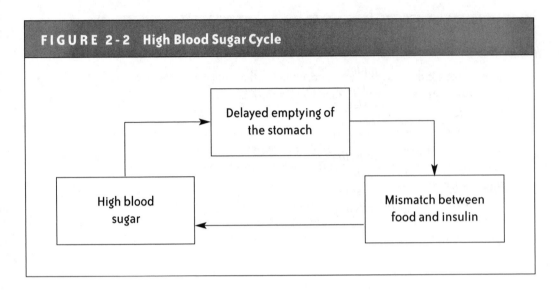

FIGURE 2-2   High Blood Sugar Cycle

How the pump can help

The pump, by giving you more stable glucose levels, can help break this vicious cycle and improve your gastroparesis symptoms. Loss of appetite isn't a concern because the pump keeps your glucose levels steady, even when gastroparesis is preventing you from eating. Furthermore, some pumps have a "square wave/extended" bolus feature (we'll talk about this later), which allows you to better match your insulin to your meal. Basically, the pump gives you better blood sugar management, which is the best way to counteract gastroparesis.

Too Good to be True? It's Okay to be Hesitant

Even though the pump offers so many benefits, many patients are hesitant to start the pump. This is completely understandable. Having a machine attached to your body can bring with it a host of emotional considerations.

To some, a pump can act as an outward symbol to the world that you have diabetes, almost like a badge (though most people mistake the pump for a pager or cell phone). Not everyone is excited to wear this badge. A lot of kids in high school and college feel a little threatened by this notion. If you're single, this can be a big emotional hurdle as well. Usually, it's a matter of taking the first step and trying the pump.

> **A patient of Dr. Wolpert's had this to say about the pump.**
>
> *"I'm not used to getting compliments on my figure, but I have for years on my sense of style. Suddenly, I have this thing sticking out of me . . . I've added an extra limb, but no sleeve to cover it. This is the biggest obstacle left to loving [the pump]. Lack of understanding the workings of the pump is part of what held me back. Some things came as a surprise to me: that doses were measured in 1/10th units; that I could safely correct for high blood sugars, even in the night; that by comparison, syringe dosing is a clunky and crude system. There is a precision in the pump solution . . . it was as much ignorance and misconceptions as emotional reasons that kept me away."*

Experiencing the benefits of the pump can help you decide whether or not it's a worthwhile trade-off.

Balancing act

Sometimes, especially at first, the pump can seem like too much effort. Occasionally, you'll just need to step back and compare the benefits and the demands—and weigh your options carefully.

Demands	Benefits
▌ Must monitor blood glucose at least 4 times a day	▌ Greater lifestyle flexibility and freedom
▌ Added responsibility of taking care of the catheter sites and pump	▌ Greater sense of control over the diabetes
▌ Extra trouble-shooting skills required	▌ Greater sense of well-being from a reduction in glucose fluctuations
▌ Can act as a visible sign of diabetes	
▌ Extra time and effort required to get started	▌ Promise of a healthier future
▌ Increased risk for Diabetic ketoacidosis	▌ Help with the dawn phenomenon
▌ Inconvenience of wearing the pump	▌ Improved hypoglycemia unawareness
▌ Catheter-site infection	▌ Improved weight control
▌ Cost	▌ Improved control during physical activity

Many people tell us, "I'm feeling pushed into trying the pump by my doctor (my parents, my friends. . .)." Only you know when the time is right, or if it will ever be right, to start pump therapy. That's your decision, and if you feel pressured into it, there's a good chance you won't give your therapy the attention and work it needs. Just remember, the people pushing you to try the pump don't have to meet up with the demands (and benefits) of the pump every day—you do.

Timing is everything

Only you will know when the time is right for you to start pump therapy. There are a variety of outside influences that can have a big impact on this decision, and eliminating the circumstances that could lead you down the path to failure is a key factor. Perhaps you're having a difficult semester in school and the stress of just trying to get good grades is hard enough as it is. The added responsibility of starting pump therapy could just be too much. Maybe you've started a new job, and all of your attention is focused on settling into the workplace. Perhaps your parents are going through a divorce. Perhaps you're going through a difficult breakup yourself. There are a thousand situations that just do not lend themselves well to starting pump therapy.

The thing to keep in mind is that starting pump therapy takes a lot of work, and the less distractions you have around you and the more stable your situation is, the better chance you have for success. You will know when the time is right. Until then, there's no need to rush your decision.

It's also important to remember that when you begin pump therapy, you are walking on a two-way street. You can "try" pump therapy and then decide that, for you, the benefits do not outweigh the drawbacks. This is not a failure; this is a thoughtful choice that you've made based on personal experience.

All Signs Point to the Pump

So, you've weighed your options and are excited about the benefits of pump therapy: tight control, flexibility, less hassle, advantages you can't get from injection therapy—the list goes on and on. Of course, you're reading this book, so there's a pretty good chance that you were already interested in starting pump therapy. What you want to know is not why to use the pump, but how to use the pump.

II

Mastering Pump Basics

3 Laying the Foundation

So we've covered all the reasons why a pump is a good idea for most people with diabetes who are insulin dependent. Now it's time to turn to the actual pump itself, cover the basics of how it works, and see how you can get the best results. Even if you've been using the pump for a little while now, covering the basics is the best way to get even better glucose control.

The first thing to keep in mind is that making the jump to pump therapy takes a good deal of patience and a little hard work. It's not an easy switch, but the long-term benefits far outweigh the initial extra effort. Try to think of beginning pump therapy not as one big leap, but rather as a series of smaller leaps over time. Many of these leaps will be forward but be prepared; some of them will almost certainly seem to point you in the wrong direction.

So let's take our first leap forward and cover the basics of how the pump works.

How the Insulin Pump Works

At the most basic level, an insulin pump is merely a small, computerized device that delivers insulin into your body. That's it—just another way to deliver your insulin.

Getting in the Mindset: Packing Your Pump Suitcase

We mentioned that starting pump therapy can seem like "making a leap," even though it's actually more like a series of small steps. Pump therapy can also be viewed as a journey—a journey to tight control over your diabetes. Like any journey, you'll need luggage to help you along the way. However, since the pump therapy journey can be as much emotional as it is physical, your pump suitcase will need to be filled with attitudes towards the journey, as opposed to clothes or supplies. Pack your pump suitcase with the following 4 concepts:

I **It will take time for things to feel natural and automatic.** When you first learned to drive a car, it took time before basic functions like turning on your blinker or just turning left felt automatic. The same is true for the pump. It will take awhile for the operations and functions of the pump to feel natural. Some of these functions may even require "tune-ups" and evaluations. Just remember that eventually, it will all fall in line.

I **You will have setbacks and times when working with your diabetes care team is frustrating.** This is a normal part of the process. Learning to think like a pancreas is no easy task. Instead of viewing these times as failures, try to look at them as potholes or detours in your journey of mastering the pump.

I **You must learn to set goals that are realistic.** You know that 1,000 miles a day in a car is an unrealistic goal. To make sure you don't get "burnt out," you'll pace yourself and do what you can in a time frame that's realistic. The same is true for pump therapy. Work with your diabetes care team to set realistic goals for glucose levels, as well as practices and behaviors.

I **You cannot control every factor dealing with your diabetes.** When you drive your car, you realize that you cannot control every other driver on the road. Sometimes you have to sit through traffic jams and navigate road repairs. In the same way, your blood glucose will do things that you will not be able to control or predict, which can be very frustrating. But this is a normal part of type 1 diabetes, and the sooner you can learn to navigate these "traffic jams" and exercise patience, the more at ease you will be with your therapy.

Mechanically, of course, a small computer works differently than a vial and syringe. Insulin pumps use a small cartridge that you fill with a fast-acting insulin from a regular vial (one type of pump offers pre-filled cartridges). The amount of insulin you put into the cartridge depends on your own personal needs.

Which Type of Pump Is Right for You?

As of summer 2002, there were 4 companies marketing pumps in the United States:

▌ **Animas (Animas R-1000)**
Telephone 1-877-937-7867
Website www.animascorp.com

▌ **Disetronic** (Disetronic Dahedi, Disetronic D-TRON, Disetronic H-TRONplus)
Telephone 1-800-280-7801
Website www.disetronic-usa.com

▌ **Medtronic MiniMed** (Medtronic MiniMed 508, Medtronic MiniMed 511 [Paradigm])
Telephone 1-800-933-3322
Website www.minimed.com

▌ **Sooil** (DANADiabecare II)
Telephone 1-866-342-2322
Website www.danapumps.com

▌ In August, 2002, a 5th company, **Deltec**, received approval from the Food and Drug Administration to market their Cozmo pump.
Telephone 1-800-826-9703
Website www.delteccozmo.com

Getting information directly from the pump companies is a good first step when researching pumps. But keep in mind, companies want to sell their products, so the information may not be completely unbiased. The recommendations of your diabetes care team will probably be the most helpful.

All pumps have similar features, but there are some differences in function you need to consider:

▌ If you have an active lifestyle and/or you've noticed a marked increase in your glucose levels after high-fat meals, a pump that has more flexible basal rate adjustments (such as the Animas R-1000, Deltec Cozmo, Disetronic D-TRON, and Medtronic MiniMed 508/511 [Paradigm] pumps) may be helpful.

▌ If you've noticed that your Humalog/Novolog doesn't adequately cover meals with slowly absorbed carbohydrates (such as pizza) or you have gastroparesis, using a pump with a square wave or extended wave bolus (such as the Animas R-1000, Deltec Cozmo, Disetronic D-TRON, and Medtronic MiniMed 508/511 [Paradigm]) may be helpful.

▌ If your work shift varies from 1 day to the next and your insulin needs vary a lot on days when you aren't working, or if you're a woman whose glucose control is affected by your menstrual cycle, a pump with multiple basal rate profiles (such as the Animas R-1000, Deltec Cozmo, Disetronic D-TRON/ Dahedi and Medtronic MiniMed 508/511 [Paradigm]) may be helpful.

▌ If you require more than 50 units of insulin a day, you may find that the Medtronic MiniMed 511 (Paradigm) doesn't hold enough insulin to meet your needs.

▌ If you have type 1 diabetes, it may be best to avoid the DANADiabecare II pump. This pump has an external "on/off" switch and has a relatively quiet alarm. There is a risk that the pump can be turned off accidentally, and if you're in a noisy environment, such as a sporting event or an aircraft, you may not hear the alarm telling you that the pump has stopped delivering insulin.

▌ The Animas R-1000 and Deltec Cozmo can deliver basal rates in increments of 0.05 units/hour, which can be helpful for people who are sensitive to insulin, or for infants and children.

▌ The Deltec Cozmo has controls that can be customized, and features such as a missed meal bolus reminder that may be helpful for children and adolescents.

The pump delivers insulin from the cartridge to your body via an *infusion set*. An infusion set consists of tubing, a catheter or cannula, and tape to secure the set to the body. The catheter is usually inserted into the tissue just beneath your skin with a guide needle, and then the needle is removed (see Chapter 7 for more on infusion sites).

So what's the aim of all this technology? To accurately mimic the activity of a healthy pancreas. Although there is only one type of insulin in the pump, it is delivered in 2 basic ways—as basal insulin and bolus doses. While we'll explain the fine-tuning of these 2 facets of pump therapy in later chapters, a brief rundown here will help you get a better grasp of the basic concepts.

As we talked about in the last chapter, the healthy pancreas releases small amounts of insulin continuously throughout the day and night (basal insulin) and larger bursts on-demand to handle sudden insulin needs (bolus doses). The basal insulin controls the body's energy supply between meals, and the bolus doses usually provide coverage for the food we eat. Several other factors affect our insulin needs, including illness, physical activity, and stress; but for the most part, these 2 basic factors are the key to understanding how pump therapy is designed to work. With a little input from you on when and how much, the pump can deliver basal insulin and bolus doses almost like a healthy pancreas. The trick is learning how to think like a pancreas.

Basal Insulin

Basal insulin has 2 basic roles in your body's daily metabolic routine. It:

- Controls your blood glucose when you're not eating.
- Keeps your liver from releasing stored glucose when it's not needed.

On the whole, basal insulin accounts for about 40–60% of your body's total insulin requirements throughout a day. Reliable basal rates allow you to benefit from the flexibility the pump can provide without running into trouble. For example, if your basal rates are set too high, you're likely to need a snack to prevent a low blood glucose reaction. Thus, establishing a steady, reliable basal rate in pump therapy is essential for good glucose control.

So how do you establish a good basal rate with your pump? We'll talk more about this in the next chapter, but for now, let's consider the basics of your basal metabolism. Your liver acts as your body's glucose reservoir, storing glucose to be released and used between meals and while you're sleeping. Basal insulin plays a vital role in letting the liver know when to release this glucose. When there's too little basal insulin, the liver releases increased amounts of glucose into the bloodstream. With more glucose pouring in and still no insulin to transport glucose into your cells, your glucose levels continue to rise higher and higher, until your body is forced to convert fat into fuel. As your body uses this fat, *ketones* are produced and enter your bloodstream. Eventually, this ketone buildup can lead to a very serious condition called *diabetic ketoacidosis* (see Chapter 9 for more on this).

So, now we understand that a key to good glucose control is establishing a basal insulin rate that lets your cells get glucose and keeps your liver from releasing glucose you can't use. Too much insulin and you run the risk of hypoglycemia. Too little insulin and your blood sugars will rise. In between these two extremes is a fine middle ground. With old insulin therapy, finding this middle ground was difficult, if not impossible. With the pump, your basal insulin can be tightly controlled to match your body's needs.

If you check your blood sugar regularly, you know that your insulin needs are not the same all through the day. Sometimes you need more insulin, sometimes less. Unfortunately, long-acting insulins, even the advanced insulins just recently introduced, have a tough time matching these varying needs. With the pump, you can adjust your basal rates to match your insulin patterns throughout the day. In the beginning, you'll probably start with a single basal rate for a 24-hour period. As you become more familiar with the pump and your control tightens, you will better tailor your basal rate. For instance, many pump users program a higher basal rate for the morning hours to counteract the *dawn phenomenon*, a period in the early morning before you wake up when your liver releases more glucose. Without this increase in the basal rate to take care of the liver, your blood glucose in the morning would be high.

You probably also notice that in addition to 24-hour fluctuations, your insulin needs vary depending on what day it is. For instance, many women require different amounts of insulin during different periods of their menstrual cycle. Many people have different insulin needs during the weekends, as opposed to the rest of the week. Your insulin requirements are always fluctuating. To help meet these requirements, some pumps allow you to program different sets of 24-hour basal patterns. You can have a basal set for the weekend and 1 for the weekday; 1 for the

*In addition to setting basal patterns for the day, some pumps allow you to program different **sets** of 24-hour patterns into the pump. See how Rick takes advantage of this capability.*

Rick is an electrician, and on weekdays he tends to be pretty active with his job. The weekends are usually his "leisure" days, often spent relaxing on the couch reading a good book or watching golf. Over time, he has learned that he has better control of his blood glucose if he uses different basal programs for the weekdays and the weekends. Instead of using the same basal rate everyday, Rick's schedule looks like this:

Monday–Friday
Midnight–2 A.M.: 0.7 units/hour
2 A.M.–8 A.M.: 0.8 units/hour
8 A.M.–Midnight: 0.7 units/hour

Saturday and Sunday
Midnight–2 A.M.: 0.7 units/hour
2 A.M.–8 A.M.: 0.9 units/hour
8 A.M.–Midnight: 0.8 units/hour

Since his insulin pump allows him to program in different basal rate programs/patterns, Rick can achieve much tighter control almost automatically.

week before you menstruate, 1 for while you're menstruating, and 1 for after. In other words, you can exactly match your basal dose for a variety of situations.

Just be prepared. Getting your basal rates exactly where they need to be is no easy task. In fact, your first few weeks or even months with the pump will be spent calibrating and adjusting your basal rates until you find the doses and patterns that are best for you. But while it may take a little elbow grease and patience on your part, getting your basal rates right in the beginning is well worth the effort. *And,* once your basal rates are programmed in, they'll keep repeating the 24-hour pattern until you tell them otherwise.

Bolus Doses

Bolus doses are quite a bit different than basal doses, and because of their "as-needed" nature, they cannot be programmed in to work automatically. Bolus doses are bursts of insulin delivered by your pump, intended to mimic the burst of insulin a pancreas releases to "cover" incoming food. With the pump, these quick bursts of insulin come in 2 main types:

1. Bolus doses taken when you eat food, otherwise known as a *food bolus.*
2. Bolus doses taken to counteract high blood glucose levels, called a *correction bolus.*

Basically, bolus doses are very similar to the injections of short-acting insulin used in traditional insulin therapy. However, the pump allows for much more flexibility than the old injection method.

Determining how much insulin to use in a bolus dose can be a little tricky. Fortunately, there are simple formulas you can use to determine how much insulin you need for certain types of situations. For a food bolus, you'll want to match up your insulin with the amount of carbohydrate you're going to be eating, since carbohydrate most dramatically affects your insulin needs. To do this, you can use your *Insulin-to-Carbohydrate Ratio* (I:Carb ratio). To determine a correction bolus, you can use another easy formula that is based on your *Sensitivity Factor* (SF). Don't worry, we'll discuss these issues more in depth in the chapters to come and show you how to use these formulas to determine your doses. Table 3-1 shows what to consider in figuring your insulin dose.

TABLE 3-1 Bolus Dose Basics		
Type of Bolus	**Used for:**	**Calculate Using:**
Food bolus	To "cover" the food you plan to eat and to prevent the rise in blood glucose caused by food	I:Carb ratio
Correction bolus	To "correct" an out of range blood glucose	SF

A Road Map for a Successful Pump Start

So now we've covered the basics and, hopefully, the pump is becoming less of a mystery to you. We know a little bit about the mechanics of the pump and have a working knowledge of basal and bolus doses. But we still have a long road ahead of us. As with any journey, it's always best to have a clearly marked road map to help you get from your starting point to your destination. So, in this section, we'll present you with a general plan to help you along your way. Keep in mind that no single plan will work for every pump user. Your method will be different to suit your own needs. Work with your diabetes care team to develop a plan that's specifically designed for you. For now, here are the fundamentals of good pump therapy.

Things you should know

The following is a list of things you should have a general knowledge of as you use the pump. It may look long right now, but as you move forward in your therapy, you'll find you pick up things rather quickly. As someone using insulin therapy, many of these concepts should already look familiar. If something on this list looks foreign to you, ask a member of your diabetes care team. You'll also find that all of these things will be covered in the course of this book.

- Pump mechanics:
  - Button-pushing
  - Filling and inserting a cartridge
  - Priming the tubing

- Infusion sites:
  - Inserting infusion sets
  - Techniques to prevent infection

- Understanding the basal and bolus aspects of insulin
- Understanding the timing and action of insulin
- Understanding the relationship between insulin action, food, physical activity, illness, and blood glucose
- Carbohydrate counting:
  - Using an I:Carb ratio

- Record keeping and analysis of data
- Troubleshooting:
  - High and low blood glucose
  - Using an SF
  - Managing unexplained hyperglycemia

- Guidelines for basal rate and bolus adjustments
- Guidelines for increased activity or exercise
- Guidelines for coming off of an insulin pump

■ Guidelines for managing illness while using an insulin pump
■ Guidelines for pump use if you need to be hospitalized
■ Traveling safely with an insulin pump

Seems like a quite a list! Fortunately, you don't need to be an expert on insulin pumps overnight. Like we said earlier, many of these concepts probably already seem familiar. Those that don't will be discussed in this book and can be explained at length by a member of your diabetes care team. How and when you acquire this knowledge will also vary from pump user to pump user. Everyone learns at a different pace, and every physician and diabetes educator has a different method for starting patients on the pump. The thing to remember is that eventually, you will need to know all of these concepts well, and you will need a physician and diabetes educator who know all of these concepts well. Knowledge is the best tool you can have when using an insulin pump. All of the technology a pump offers can be wasted if you don't know how to use it properly.

The road map

How and when you acquire the information and knowledge you'll need to be successful with the pump is almost as important as the knowledge itself. If you try to learn it all at once, there's a good chance that you'll get overwhelmed. Learn certain aspects at the wrong time, and you'll be unprepared to move forward. For instance, if you know how to adjust your basal rates around activity (a relatively advanced concept), but don't know how to change your infusion site, you won't be prepared for pump therapy. Luckily, pump-related knowledge is very organic and will evolve naturally, with the more complicated aspects building off of the simpler concepts you learn at first. In other words, you'll need to know the basics to understand the more intense therapy. If it all looks a little overwhelming, just think how much you knew when you started insulin therapy, and compare that to how much you know now! Each little tidbit of knowledge you picked up, or skill you mastered, happened over time and built on what you already knew. The same will happen with pump therapy. Just be patient and the rest will happen.

Table 3-2 represents a typical pump-related knowledge flow. Consider this your road map, marking where you need to be as you travel towards your pump therapy destination. Once again, this may be differ-

	TABLE 3-2 A Typical Road Map to Beginning Insulin Pump Therapy	
Time Frame	**What You Should Expect to Understand or Learn:**	**What You Should Be Doing:**
Weeks to months before beginning pump therapy	▌ The relationship of food, exercise, and illness to blood glucose levels ▌ The action profiles of insulin ▌ Advanced carbohydrate counting	▌ Carbohydrate counting ▌ Regularly checking blood glucose a minimum of 4–6 times per day ▌ Keeping food, insulin, activity, and blood glucose records ▌ Analyzing your records
One to 2 weeks before beginning pump therapy	▌ Pump mechanics ▌ Infusion set insertion ▌ The concepts of basal/bolus doses in pump delivery ▌ Working knowledge of using I:Carb ratios and insulin SF to calculate bolus doses ▌ Basic troubleshooting of high and low blood glucose while on a pump ▌ How much insulin to take the day before and the day of start	▌ Continuing with the tasks above, but keeping hypothetical records calculating bolus doses as if you were on the pump ▌ Reading the manual and watching the video that comes with your insulin pump ▌ Practicing pump mechanics ▌ Practicing infusion set insertion
Day of pump start	▌ A firm grasp of troubleshooting highs ▌ When to check for ketones ▌ When to take an injection ▌ Who to call for technical and clinical assistance	▌ Increasing the frequency of blood glucose checks to 8–10 times per day (temporarily) ▌ Keeping specific pump logs
One to 2 weeks after pump start	▌ Troubleshooting ▌ Plans for managing blood glucose around physical activity	▌ Basal rate evaluations ▌ Keeping in contact with pump trainer and/or MD
Two weeks to several months after pump start	▌ Effects of various foods on blood glucose ▌ Variable bolus options ▌ Multiple basal rates during the day and multiple-day profiles	▌ Possibly continuing basal rate evaluations ▌ Bolus dose evaluations

ent for you and your particular situation, but as a general rule of thumb, it's an adequate starting point.

A lot to learn, to be sure. Luckily, you won't have to learn it all on your own. As you begin your pump therapy, your team of diabetes care professionals will be there every step of the way to help you gain the knowledge you need. Most of this teaching will come in the form of appointments and meetings with these professionals. Following is a list of what you can expect to encounter at these various meetings.

- **Pre-pump interview:** This is a time for you to meet with a diabetes educator, or pump trainer, to talk about the benefits and challenges of pump therapy as they relate to your situation. It gives you both a chance to consider if using the pump is the right decision and to agree upon an education plan tailored for your needs. It's also a good time for you to learn about the different types of pumps and explore your options.

- **Pre-pump education:** This may consist of various appointments and topics depending on your needs. It really depends on what you and your diabetes care team feel you need to know more about before starting the pump. For instance, if you need education in carb counting, you may meet with a Registered Dietitian to help you move forward. Check the list of things you should know and the chart above. If there's anything on either of those that you don't feel comfortable with, talk to a member of your diabetes care team about how you can get up to speed.

- **Saline trial:** This is a common approach to getting you comfortable with the pump, though not all pump educators and physicians will go this route. Basically, you wear a pump like you would normally, using saline (salt water) instead of insulin. This is usually done a few days to a week before you plan to start the pump and incorporates the mechanics and physical aspects of the pump into your normal routine. You'll learn how the pump works (buttons, cartridges, infusion sets, etc.) and how to comfortably wear the pump in a variety of situations. Be prepared. This can tend to be a difficult week, as you're not only learning how to live with the pump, but also maintaining your regular insulin regimen. Rest assured that the extra work is worth the effort. Once you start using the pump to manage your diabetes, being familiar with the mechanics will allow you to focus on your blood glucose and not the buttons you push to keep it under control. Even if you don't undergo a saline trial, you should spend the first couple of weeks before you start pump therapy playing with the pump, watching the video, reading the manual, and just getting yourself familiar with how it works.

- ■ **Insulin start:** The day you begin pumping! Expect to review some pump mechanics and focus on troubleshooting and record keeping. You'll probably also cover the process involved in basal rate evaluations. Be sure to talk with your diabetes care team about how much insulin you should take the day before and the day of your pump start.

- ■ **Follow-up:** These appointments will vary depending on your needs and the methods of your diabetes care team. During the first few days, expect a lot of phone conversations, faxes, and emails concerning blood glucose levels and initial changes in dosage. Over the next few weeks and months, there will be several in-person visits with your health care team to go over the basics, start learning more advanced aspects of pump therapy, and begin the fine-tuning process.

Remember that the easiest and most effective way to learn is to ask questions. Don't be intimidated by members of your diabetes care team. They are there to help you and want to make the transition to the pump as easy as possible. The old adage that "there's no such thing as a stupid question" holds true here—maybe even more so since it's your health that's on the line!

Eye Care Before You Start Pump Therapy

A number of studies—most importantly, the Diabetes Control and Complications Trial (DCCT)—have clearly shown that there are numerous long-term benefits to be gained by tightening your glucose control. Overall, your risk of complications down the road is drastically reduced. This includes retinopathy (diabetic eye disease).

Strangely, however, there's a chance that if you already have retinopathy, your condition could actually get worse during the first year or so of intensive therapy. If your A1C levels are very high in the beginning and then rapidly reduce, you run the highest risk of this deterioration. Keep in mind that the long-term benefits of tight diabetes control far outweigh the risks of worsening retinopathy in the early stages of intensive therapy. Also keep in mind that this risk for worsening can occur whether diabetes control is intensified by either multiple injections or the insulin pump. In fact, none of the people studied in the DCCT who suffered from worsened retinopathy early on developed any serious loss of vision.

The lesson to be learned from this is simple—always have a dilated eye exam before you start any intensive therapy, including pump therapy. You should also talk to your ophthalmologist (eye doctor) about whether or not you should have more frequent eye checks once you start tightening your control. (See Appendix A for a sample letter to your ophthalmologist.)

Keeping Your Expectations Realistic

As you start pump therapy, you're probably going to feel a breadth of emotions, running the gamut from nervous to anxious to relieved. More than likely, you'll also be excited about the new freedom and ease you plan to get from your pump. There were probably some specific features that drew you to the pump and you can't wait to take advantage of them. And you're right to be excited. Just be sure to keep things in perspective. The pump is a great tool, but it is not a miracle device that will magically give you perfect glucose control. The pump is still just a method of delivering insulin, and it has its own set of limitations.

Unfortunately, it's easy to be deceived. The first few days on the pump will sometimes seem absolutely perfect, and controlling your blood glucose may seem easier than ever before. This is what a lot of pump users refer to as the *pump honeymoon*—those first few days of bliss when it seems that absolutely nothing can go wrong. Soon, however, the frustration starts to set in as out-of-range glucose readings start popping up, and it's easy to start thinking your therapy is actually getting worse. More than likely, you're just checking more often than usual, and these off-target readings may have already been there and you're just now seeing them. But still, you can go from elated to frustrated pretty quickly.

Always try to remember that pump therapy is just a tool to help you get better control over your diabetes—nothing more, nothing less. It's not perfect, but it's one of the best tools we have.

4

Getting Your Basal Rates on Track

By now you're probably well aware of what a basal rate is and how it operates in your body; it provides the background coverage you need to keep operating throughout the day and night. Sounds simples, doesn't it? Well, you'll soon discover that finding a basal rate that works right for you can be deceivingly difficult. Basal rates may not require the constant attention that bolus doses do, but determining a pattern that matches your needs can take months of fine-tuning and evaluation.

Start with Your Total Daily Dose

One of the first steps in insulin pump therapy (after educating yourself about the pump and how it works) will be to translate your current insulin regimen into basal rates and bolus doses. Keep in mind that this will be an *estimate*. As you move along, these beginning rates and doses will be fine-tuned, partially by you and partially by your physician or diabetes educator. When you start, however, a member of your diabetes care team will set your initial dose. **DO NOT** try to estimate your initial basal rate and bolus doses on your own. This section will give you an overview of the most common methods to estimate these doses from you current insulin regimen.

The first step in estimating your pump basal rates is determining your Total Daily Dose (TDD) of insulin. Start by considering how much insulin you use now. Simply add up the average number of units you take in 1 day, making sure to include all types of insulin you are currently taking. Since the pump tends to use insulin more efficiently than injection therapy, you will need to lower this amount to determine your pump levels. Generally, reducing your pre-pump TDD by 25% will tell you what your TDD will be with the pump.

A Simple Formula for Determining Your TDD on the Pump

Current TDD   − 25% = Estimate of TDD on insulin pump
(pre-pump TDD)   (pump TDD)

Of course there will be deviations from this rule. There are several things your physician will take into account when determining your beginning TDD on the pump. For example, if you tend to have consistently high blood glucose, your physician will probably lower your TDD less than 25%. If, on the other hand, you have problems with hypoglycemia, it would probably be wise to reduce your TDD by more than 25%. It really depends on where you are in your current insulin therapy and where you would like to be down the road.

There are other methods for determining an initial TDD for the pump, as well. One way is to multiply your weight in kilograms by 0.7 (to figure out your weight in kilograms, divide your weight in pounds by 2.2). For example, a man who weighs 212 pounds, would divide 212 by 2.2 to determine his weight in kilograms (96.36 kg), and then multiply this number by 0.7 to get 67.45 as his TDD. Rounding this down to 67, he gets a general estimate of his insulin needs as an adult.

If the numbers you get from the weight method don't quite jive with the numbers you get from the current TDD adjustment method, your physician will probably go with the lower number to be safe. As you start pump therapy, avoiding low blood sugar reactions takes priority over extremely tight control.

> **Remember!**
>
> **Your physician will determine your initial insulin pump doses.**

Your Initial Basal Rates

Now we know about how much insulin you will be using a day. But how much of this will go to basal insulin and how much will go towards bolus doses? A good place to start with your basal rate is to assume that 50% of your TDD will be used for basal insulin, with the remaining 50% going towards your bolus doses. This is, of course, a rough estimate and will more than likely change as you begin to adjust your rates. But it's a good starting point.

As you move forward with your therapy, you will probably take advantage of having multiple basal rates for the day (and with some pumps, for the week). But to begin with, it's probably best to start with a single basal rate and move on from there. Pumps administer basal doses in hourly increments, so you'll need to know how much insulin you'll need an hour to determine your starting basal rate. To calculate this number, simply take your new pump TDD and cut it in half. This will tell you how much insulin you'll need for your daily basal rate. Then, simply divide this number by 24 to find your hourly basal rate.

> **Formula for Determining Your Initial Basal Rate**
>
> Pump TDD ÷ 2 = Estimated daily basal needs
>
> Estimated ÷ 24 = Basal rate daily basal in units/hour needs

> **Caution!**
>
> If you do not recognize symptoms of low blood glucose, or if you experience relatively wide blood glucose fluctuations, it's wise to take less insulin than initial basal rate estimates indicate. Remember, avoiding low blood sugar reactions takes precedence over extremely tight control.

Evaluating Your Initial Basal Rates

Not long after you start pump therapy using your initial basal rate, you'll probably realize that one constant rate isn't going to provide the tight control you were looking for. Now it's time to evaluate your initial rate and begin to make adjustments. This is the first big step (made up of many smaller steps) towards optimizing your control with pump therapy. Once your basal rates are established, you can begin to work on the tricky part of pump therapy—evaluating and fine-tuning your bolus doses.

As you begin checking your basal rates, there are some things you should keep in mind. The following list details some guidelines for ensuring your evaluations are accurate and consistent.

- The first time frame you evaluate should be the overnight basal rate. This is most often the time frame that needs adjusting.
- Typically, the same results should occur at least *twice* before you consider it a pattern and make adjustments to your basal rate. However, if your blood glucose is dropping dramatically during an evaluation, it's wise to change the rate without confirming a pattern.
- Your blood glucose should be between 100 and 150 mg/dl before you proceed with an evaluation.
- During the day of an evaluation, you should not exercise, eat high-fat meals, or drink alcohol. Doing so could compromise the accuracy of the evaluation.
- The last meal before you begin an evaluation should be easily matched to bolus doses. In other words, your bolus doses should accurately match your food intake so you have an accurate starting point from which to begin your evaluation. Low-fat foods are a good choice for this meal.
- Stop your evaluation if your blood glucose drops below or rises above your target range. Treat these fluctuations as you normally would. You may still get valuable information from these experiences.
- Do not plan an evaluation if you have had any severe low blood glucose reactions earlier that day.
- Do not plan a basal rate evaluation if you are sick or under unusual stress. These situations tend to increase insulin requirements and are not the best times to run an evaluation.
- Basal evaluations can generally begin 4–5 hours after your last bolus. The bolus will usually be used up by then.

■ During an evaluation, you should check your blood glucose levels every 1–2 hours. For the overnight time frame, check your levels before bedtime, midnight, between 2 and 3 A.M., and upon waking.

■ It is very important that you keep accurate and detailed records so your physician and/or diabetes educator can help you evaluate the information and assess your basal rates. See Chapter 9, "Keeping Track and Tracking Trouble," for some sample insulin pump record sheets that you can model your records after.

So now that you have some guidelines to keep in mind as you evaluate your basal rates, you're ready to move onto your evaluations. Table 4-1 details the steps you need to take as you evaluate your basal

TABLE 4-1 Step-by-Step Basal Rate Evaluation		
Time Frames and Directions	**When to Check Blood Glucose**	**Evaluating Your Results**
Overnight: ▮ Eat an early dinner (don't forget your meal bolus!) ▮ Eat no food afterwards ▮ Begin evaluation at bedtime	❏ 4–5 hours after dinner bolus ❏ Bedtime ❏ Midnight ❏ 2–3 A.M. ❏ Upon waking	Basal rates are correct if blood glucose (BG) does not increase or decrease more than 30–40 mg/dl during evaluation. **If BG increases:** Your basal rate needs to be increased for this time period. **If BG decreases:** Your basal rate needs to be decreased for this time period.
Breakfast-time: ▮ Check your BG upon waking and begin evaluation if BG is between 100 and 150 mg/dl ▮ Skip breakfast ▮ Eat no food until lunch	❏ Every 1–2 hours upon waking until lunch	Same as above. (*Continued*)

TABLE 4-1 Step-by-Step Basal Rate Evaluation (*Continued*)		
Time Frames and Directions	**When to Check Blood Glucose**	**Evaluating Your Results**
Lunch-time: ▌ Check blood glucose before lunch time and begin evaluation if BG is between 100 and 150 mg/dl ▌ Skip lunch ▌ Eat no food until dinner	❏ 4 hours after breakfast ❏ Every 1–2 hours until dinner	Same as above.
Dinner-time: ▌ Check blood glucose before dinner time and begin evaluation if BG is between 100 and 150 mg/dl ▌ Skip dinner ▌ Eat a bedtime snack or a late dinner and end the evaluation there if you desire	❏ 4 hours after lunch ❏ Every 1–2 hours until dinner or snack	Same as above.

If your basal rate is too *high*, your blood glucose will *drop* during a basal rate evaluation. If your basal rate is too *low*, your blood glucose will *rise* during a basal rate evaluation.

rates. Remember that you should **NEVER** evaluate all of these time periods on the same day.

As you can see, there's a lot to consider! You probably also recognize that evaluating your basal rates is no easy task. You might even be asking yourself how the pump is supposed to be making your life easier. Just remember; the extra steps you take in the beginning of pump therapy reap long-lasting results. Plus, all of this extra effort in the beginning doesn't have to be done at once. Pace yourself. Do what you can, and take breaks when you need to. Fit evaluations into your schedule when it's convenient. If you can't do an overnight evaluation today, but a morning evaluation will easily fit into your daily routine, do a morning evaluation. There may even be times when you didn't plan on doing an evaluation, but the situation presented itself. For example, there's a day when you're too busy to take a lunch break. If you just do a few extra blood glucose checks . . . voila, you've just completed an afternoon basal rate evaluation!

Using the Information You've Gathered— Adjusting Your Basal Rates

So now you know how to collect information from your evaluations. This information is the starting point for tightening your control with the pump. At first, you'll want to work with your physician and/or diabetes educator to see what changes you need to make. As you gain experience, you'll be able to make some of these changes on your own.

Just like with the evaluations, there are some guidelines you need to keep in mind as you begin to adjust your rates. Remember, the first few months will be a period of constant evaluation and adjustment. It may seem like a lot, but if you keep certain things in mind and follow some of the basic "rules" we've presented in this book, everything will fall into place.

Guidelines for adjusting basal rates

- Fluctuations of more than 30–40 mg/dl during an evaluation indicate a need to adjust your basal rates.
- It is best to see a repeating trend before making a basal change.
- Make small changes, typically 0.05–0.10 units/hour.
- You should increase or decrease your basal rate at least 1–2 hours before your blood glucose begins to rise or fall as indicated by your evaluations. It takes a little while for a basal rate change to begin to have an impact.
- Make one change at a time, and then reevaluate that time frame.
- **Check with your physician and/or diabetes educator before you change your basal rate.** Eventually, they may expect you to make your own adjustments.
- **Remember, the goal is to find the basal rates that work best most of the time.** Don't expect perfection!

The bulk of your evaluating and adjusting will take place when you start pump therapy, but periodic evaluations and adjustments after your initial therapy are necessary as well. Like we said before, this may sound like a lot to take in at first. Lots of "rules," lots of guidelines, lots of procedures to follow. All of this information is important, and all of it applies to your therapy. But of all the guidelines we have introduced, the following 2 are probably the most important in relation to basal rates:

- When evaluating your basal rates, minimize the factors that affect your basal insulin requirements, such as exercise, high-fat foods, and alcohol (See Chapter 10 for more). If you keep this in mind, everything else should fall into place.
- When adjusting your basal rates, your goal is to find the basal rates that work best most of the time. Try to find the *best* fit and keep in mind that there is no *perfect* fit.

Using Multiple Basal Rate Programs

Many pumps allow you to program in more than one basal rate profile. Using this function allows you to use different sets of 24-hour programs whenever you like. This is very helpful for people who have different activity levels throughout the week, women during different stages of their menstrual cycle, or people who work different shifts at their job.

Since this function varies from pump to pump, there's no standard set of rules you can follow. Learning about your specific pump from the materials the pump manufacturer provides will get you up to speed on the mechanics. As for guidelines you should follow when deciding on multiple programs; well, that's up to you and your insulin needs. Using the information you obtain from your evaluations, you and your diabetes educator and/or physician will be able to determine what rates at what times will work best for you.

At first, you'll probably stick with one basal rate program. It will take awhile just to find one program that fits your needs. But by keeping detailed records of your diabetes management, you'll be able to determine alternate programs later on down the road.

When to reassess your basal rates

Although the bulk of your evaluating/adjusting happens when you first start pump therapy, there will be other times when you'll need to revisit the evaluating process. The following reasons may lead you to further basal rate evaluations from time to time.

- Change in body weight
- Change in everyday activity level
- Change in job
- Pregnancy

■ Just a general sense that your rates aren't working as well as they should

> **What would you do?**
>
> Beth completes 3 breakfast-time basal evaluations on 3 consecutive days. She finds that on 2 days, her blood glucose clearly trended up more than 30–40 mg/dl. On 1 day, her blood glucose trended down a little bit. She thinks about her activity levels during the 3 days and decides that there wasn't any noticeable difference. She feels that, in general, her blood glucose tends to "run a bit high" in the early part of the day.
>
> Working off of this, she decides to adjust her basal rate up slightly and then reevaluate.

Other things to think about

There are a couple of additional things to consider as you are evaluating your basal rates.

■ Keep in mind that, unfortunately, blood glucose meters and the testing process are not perfect. Since meters are calibrated differently, it is imperative that you use the **same** type of meter while doing a basal evaluation. Furthermore, there is evidence that alternate site (i.e., the forearm) monitoring can be misleading at times, so while your doing basal rate evaluations, it would probably be best to stick to fingersticks.

■ Second, don't get too picky with isolated numbers. It's best to look for trends.

■ Finally, remember that this is not a perfect science! Without acknowledging this, evaluating basal rates can become a never-ending task. Your goal should be to find a basal profile that works for you **most** of the time.

So there you have it—a step-by-step approach to getting your basal rates up to speed. It may seem like a lot at first (and it is!), but the effort is well worth the results. Once you get your basal rates set, you'll find that you'll rarely have to bother with them. To some degree, they take care of themselves. But getting them right *is* important. Having your basal rates on track is absolutely essential for the aspect of pump therapy that will require constant attention—your bolus doses.

5 Figuring Out Your Bolus Doses

First Things First

It may seem hard to believe now, but in some respects, figuring out your basal rates is the easy part. Once your basal rates are fine-tuned, you rarely have to think about them on a day-to-day basis unless you experience unexpected high or low blood sugars during periods without food. You get the ball rolling and the pump pretty much takes it from there. Bolus doses, on the other hand, require quite a bit more daily consideration.

Unfortunately, it's easy to get discouraged by all of the attention and work that go into bolus doses. Once again, you may start asking yourself, "How is this supposed to be easier?" The thing to keep in mind is that ease is not the only advantage of the pump. Flexibility is also a benefit you reap when you make the switch to the pump. If you look at it this way, the extra attention you pay to bolus doses is actually a positive thing, the trade-off being more freedom in your therapy and lifestyle.

Estimating your initial bolus dose

Looking back to when you estimated your initial basal rate, you'll see that approximately half of your Total Daily Dose

(TDD) was reserved for your bolus doses. This is just a rough estimate and may not actually correspond to the amount of insulin you use for boluses. Your actual bolus doses will be matched to the food you eat and your glucose levels, rather than just being arbitrarily spread out throughout the day. In other words, your bolus doses will be calculated using your I:Carb ratio and your SF. Just like with basal rates, there are various ways to estimate your initial I:Carb ratio and SF bolus doses.

Estimating your initial SF

The SF is used to decide how much insulin you take to correct a high blood glucose. Simply put, the number you get for your SF is how many milligrams per deciliter 1 unit of insulin will lower your blood glucose. For example, if your SF turns out to be 40, then a bolus of 1 unit of insulin will generally (with "generally" being the key word) lower your blood glucose 40 mg/dl. Keep in mind that like a lot of things in the world of diabetes, this is not set in stone. If your SF is 40, there will be times when a bolus of 1 unit will lower your blood glucose about 50 mg/dl; other times it might lower it 30 mg/dl. There are always variations.

So how do you determine your initial SF? Actually, it's pretty easy. An SF is commonly calculated using the "1500-rule." (You may also have heard of the "1800-rule." In practice, since this rule is just used to calculate an initial SF that will later be refined, it doesn't matter which you use.) The "1500-rule" states that an SF can be estimated by dividing 1500 by your TDD (that's the entire TDD, not just the half estimated for bolus doses). For simplicity, the result can be rounded to the nearest multiple of 10.

> **Example Calculation of an SF Using the "1500-rule"**
>
> Pre-pump TDD = 72 units
> Pump TDD estimate = 54 units (72 units − 25%)
> 1500 ÷ 54 = 28 . . . round to 30
> **SF = 30**

Remember, the SF is just an estimate! The "1500-rule" is not based on "hard" science; it's just a practical way to estimate a general starting point. After that, it's a matter of practice, experience, and evaluation to see if this SF is the right one for you, or if it needs to be modified.

Most pump users also benefit from more than 1 SF. For example, you may need a different bedtime SF to help prevent hypoglycemia while you sleep. Likewise, a higher SF might be needed for boluses administered right before you exercise, or you may need a lower SF when your glucose is very high. As you've probably realized, the higher SF translates to lower bolus doses, since an increase in sensitivity (responsiveness) to insulin means it will take less insulin to lower your blood glucose. Conversely, the lower SF translates to bigger bolus doses, since a decrease in sensitivity to insulin means it will take more insulin to lower your blood glucose.

Estimating your initial I:Carb ratio

An I:Carb ratio is basically a way to simply express how many grams of carbohydrate 1 unit of insulin will cover. There's a good chance you're already using an I:Carb ratio. If this is the case, you may start pump therapy using the same I:Carb ratio you're already using. This is really at the discretion of your physician and/or diabetes educator. More than likely, you'll find that the I:Carb ratio you're using for injection therapy won't work as well for your pump therapy and that some modifications will be necessary.

If you're not using an I:Carb ratio, don't worry; there are a couple of easy ways to determine one. You may work with a Registered Dietitian (RD) who can help you determine an I:Carb ratio from food, insulin, and blood glucose records that you keep (actually, no matter how you determine your I:Carb ratio, it's best to consult with an RD). Another method is by using the "450-rule." (Just like with the "1500-rule," there are variations on this rule, most notably the "500-rule." Once again, since these are just initial estimates, either rule should work fine). This rule states that your ratio can be determined by dividing 450 by your pump TDD.

Just like with the SF, rounding the numbers to make calculations easier is perfectly fine. These initial settings are merely starting points that will be evaluated and refined as you move forward in your therapy. Thus, if your calculations yield a 1:11 ratio, you'd probably be safe going with a 1:10 ratio to make figuring out your boluses easier.

Example Calculation for an I:Carb Using the "450-rule"

Pre-pump TDD = 63 units
Pump TDD estimate = 47 units (63 units − 25%)
450 ÷ 47 = 9.6…rounded to 10
I:Carb = 1:10

So now you have the means to figure out your initial SF and I:Carb ratios. You have a starting point from which to move forward—the block of marble from which you can carve the accurate and tight control you had imagined. But an SF and an I:Carb ratio are just tools, and like any tool, they're no good unless you know how to use them. In the next section, we'll show you how to use the SF and I:Carb ratio to calculate your bolus doses.

Using Your SF and I:Carb Ratio to Calculate Bolus Doses

As we've mentioned before, there are two types of boluses you will use with the pump—the bolus you take when you eat, which we call your *food bolus*, and the bolus you use to correct high blood sugar, which we call your *correction bolus*. In the last section, we discussed the tools you will use to determine each of these boluses—your SF and I:Carb ratio. But these are not the only factors determining your bolus doses. In this section, we will discuss what you need to consider when calculating a bolus dose. This includes:

- The amount of carbohydrate you plan to eat.
- The amount of carbohydrate that is "covered" by 1 unit of insulin—your I:Carb ratio.
- Your blood glucose at the time you're planning to bolus.
- How much 1 unit of insulin will lower your blood glucose—your SF.
- The length of time since your last bolus.
- Your target blood glucose.

Food bolus

There are 3 energy-yielding nutrients in the food you eat—protein, fat, and carbohydrate. Of the 3, carbohydrate has the greatest effect on your blood glucose. So, the first step in determining your food bolus is to learn how to accurately estimate how many grams of carbohydrate you plan to eat. We'll talk about carbohydrate counting at length later in the book; so for now, we'll just assume you know the carb counts in the food you're eating. Using just this number, and your I:Carb ratio, you now have everything you need to determine your food bolus.

When we talked about how to determine your I:Carb ratio above, you probably wondered what the numbers you were working with meant. Basically, this ratio tells you how much carbohydrate **1** unit of

Calculating Your Food Bolus

The formula for figuring out your food bolus is relatively straightforward. Just take the number of grams of carbohydrates you're going to eat, and divide it by the 2nd number in your I:Carb ratio. Expressed another way, it looks like the following:

Carbohydrate grams ÷ X = number of insulin units to bolus

(X = *the 2nd number of your I:Carb ratio*)

Example

Janet plans to eat 25 g of carbohydrate at lunch. Her I:Carb ratio is 1:15. So, to figure out how much she needs to bolus to cover her meal, she simply divides 25 by 15.

25 g of carb ÷ 15 = 1.7 units of bolus

Using this formula, Janet can see that she needs to bolus 1.7 units of insulin to cover the food she plans to eat.

rapid-acting insulin will cover. The ratio will always be expressed as 1:X, with the numeral 1 representing a unit of insulin, and X being the amount of carbohydrate this unit will cover. So, if your I:Carb ratio is 1:10, you will need 1 unit of insulin to cover every 10 grams of carbs you eat.

Each I:Carb ratio will be different from person to person. Generally the ratio is related to how sensitive (responsive) you are to insulin. If you're relatively sensitive to insulin, 1 unit of insulin is going to cover more carbohydrates than usual, and the second number of your I:Carb ratio will be higher than most. To put it another way, someone with an I:Carb of 1:20 will need to bolus less insulin than someone with an I:Carb of 1:10 to cover the same amount of carbohydrates. In fact, they'll only need to bolus half as much.

In addition to variations from person to person, I:Carb ratios may also be different for a single person at different times of the day. For instance, you may benefit from using a different I:Carb ratio for your evening meals than the one you use for breakfast. We'll talk more about this in Chapter 10.

Correction bolus

If we lived in a perfect world, there'd be no need for a correction bolus. Your basal insulin would perfectly match your insulin needs, while your

Calculating Your Correction Boluses

Like we said before, calculating your correction bolus is pretty easy. Simply subtract your Target Blood Glucose (BG) from your Current BG, and then divide that number by your SF.

$$\text{(Current BG} - \text{Target BG)} \div \text{SF} = \text{Correction Bolus}$$

The same formula works for both high blood glucose corrections and low blood glucose corrections, as you'll see from the examples below.

Example of correction bolus for high blood sugar

Janet checks her blood glucose and sees that her Current BG is 253 mg/dl. Her Target BG is well below that, at 120 mg/dl. She has an SF of 70. To figure out what her Correction Bolus should be, she first subtracts her Target BG of 120 from her Current BG of 253 to get the number 133. She then divides this number by her SF of 70. From this, she gets her Correction Bolus of 1.9 units of insulin. The same steps can be shown as follows:

$$\text{Current BG} = 253 \text{ mg/dl}$$
$$\text{Target BG} = 120 \text{ mg/dl}$$
$$\text{SF} = 70$$
$$(253 - 120) \div 70 = (133) \div 70 = 1.9 \text{ units of insulin*}$$

*If it is mealtime, Janet will add this to her food bolus.

Example of correction bolus for low blood sugar

Another time, Janet checks her blood sugar again and sees that it has fallen well below her Target BG of 120 mg/dl, to a Current BG of 68 mg/dl. Using the same SF as before (70), she does the following to figure out her Correction Bolus. Once again, she subtracts her Target BG from her Current BG; only now, since her Current BG is lower than her Target BG, she's going to get a negative number: −52. She then divides this by her SF of 70 to get −0.74, which she can just round up to −0.7 units of insulin to make things easy.

Shown another way:

$$\text{Current BG} = 68 \text{ mg/dl}$$
$$\text{Target BG} = 120 \text{ mg/dl}$$
$$\text{SF} = 70$$
$$(68 - 120) \div 70 = (-52) \div 70 = -0.7 \text{ units of insulin (rounded up)}$$

Since Janet's final number is a negative number, this means she will need to use much *less* insulin as a correction. During meal or snack time, this isn't much of a problem—she can just *subtract* this much insulin from her food bolus to even things out. However, if she wasn't planning on eating, how can she take a negative bolus? Well, she can't. She'll need to eat some fast-acting carbohydrate that will get her blood glucose levels back to normal.

food boluses would accurately matched the carbohydrates you were taking in. Unfortunately, we don't live in a perfect world, and pump therapy is not a perfect therapy. As such, the correction bolus is a very important part of your new therapy.

What happens when your blood glucose is too high before a meal? Even if your food bolus is accurate, you're going to end up with high blood sugar after your food bolus runs its course. What happens if it's too low? A bolus that matches up with your food is going to bring your blood glucose back down below your target range. This is where the correction bolus comes in.

To get your blood glucose back to your target range, you'll need to "correct" your levels by bolusing extra insulin if your blood glucose is high. On the other hand, if your blood glucose is too low, you may need to "correct" this glucose by taking a smaller than usual food bolus if it is meal or snack time. Another plan is to eat some carbohydrate right away to bring up your blood glucose.

Just like with your food bolus, calculating your correction bolus is pretty simple. All you need to know is your target blood glucose range and your SF. After that, you're just a few calculations away!

Correction Bolus—Things to Think About

When to correct?

Most correction boluses take place at meal or snack time, which makes sense—this is usually when you check your blood glucose. This also makes correction boluses much easier to calculate. If your blood glucose is running high, just tack the correction bolus onto your food bolus. If, however, your blood glucose is running low, you could simply subtract your correction bolus from your food bolus. But remember, this may not always be the best option. For example, if you eat slowly, you will be eating a relatively high-fat meal, or your blood glucose is falling rapidly, the food may not raise your blood glucose fast enough for the "correction" to your food bolus to be effective. The best method for correcting low blood glucose is to eat some fast-acting carbohydrate and get your blood glucose levels back to normal before bolusing your food dose.

Not all correction boluses take place at mealtime, however. Sometimes, a correction bolus is called for between meals. A random blood glucose check may reveal that your levels are above or below your target ranges. At times like these, your first instinct might be to just bolus a correction based simply on your SF. But there's more to consider. When bolusing a correction, you must always keep in mind the size and timing of your last bolus.

Your last bolus

Correction bolus doses are rarely independent of your other bolus doses, and figuring a correction without factoring in your other doses can lead to some problems. The biggest problem is overlapping doses. For example, say you correct a high blood glucose by taking a correction bolus at 10 A.M. Sometime around noon, you get ready to eat lunch. You check your blood sugar and even though it has decreased some, it's still higher than your target. Your first instinct might be to add another correction bolus to your food bolus. However, the "tail" of the first bolus is still acting a bit, and an additional bolus could overlap with the first bolus, leaving you with a low blood sugar (Fig. 5-1).

How much overlap you're liable to get varies depending on the type of insulin in your pump, the size of the bolus, and your individual response. Following are the general action times of both Humalog/Novolog and regular insulin:

- **Humalog/Novolog:** In general, you can expect about 1/2 of a Humalog/Novolog bolus to be used up after 2 hours. In other words, after 2 hours, 1/2 of your bolus is still at work. Usually, a

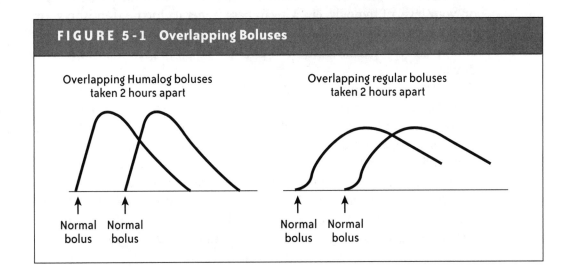

FIGURE 5-1   Overlapping Boluses

Overlapping Humalog boluses
taken 2 hours apart

Normal   Normal
bolus   bolus

Overlapping regular boluses
taken 2 hours apart

Normal   Normal
bolus   bolus

Humalog/Novolog bolus will run its course between 3 and 5 hours. As you move forward with your therapy, you'll be able to better pinpoint your own response. Fine-tuned basal rates also help this process.

■ **Regular:** Expect 1/2 of a bolus of regular insulin to be used after about 3 hours. In fact, a bolus of regular insulin may still be having some impact 6–8 hours later!

Keeping these insulin action profiles in mind will help you avoid a common cause of hypoglycemia—overtreating high blood glucose. Before you bolus a corrective dose, pause to consider if your previous bolus is still at work in your system. If you're impatient about getting the glucose down (and why shouldn't you be?) and you're compelled to take a second dose, play it safe and bolus less than the full calculated dose. We'll talk more about this in Chapter 10.

A word about target blood glucose

As you've probably noticed, target blood glucose levels play a very important part in determining your bolus doses. Since you're probably already familiar with the concept of target blood glucose, as well as your own values, we won't discuss this at length. However, there are some things to keep in mind when considering target blood glucose values in relation to pump therapy and, in particular, bolus doses.

Target values are generally thought of as ranges. Most people have a range of 80–120 mg/dl. Your value may be higher than this, depending on your level of hypoglycemia awareness, general glucose trends in your body, and other factors (Table 5-1). With the help of your physician and/or diabetes educator, the best possible target range can be pinned down.

While these ranges make it easier to attain healthy glucose levels, they also make it difficult to calculate bolus doses. How do you add or subtract from a "range" of numbers? To simplify this operation, find the number in the middle of your target blood glucose range and use this in your bolus dose calculations. For example, if your target range is 80–120 mg/dl, you would use "100" in your calculations.

And always remember that no person, no matter how diligent, can keep his or her blood glucose values in their target range all the time. Getting as close as you possibly can at all times should be your aim.

TABLE 5-1 Blood Glucose Goals for People with Diabetes			
Target Blood Glucose (individualized)	Normal (mg/dl) (whole blood-capillary)	Normal (mg/dl) (plasma values)	Goal (mg/dl) (whole blood-capillary)
Non-pregnancy			
Average before meals	<100	<110	80–120
2 hours after meals		<140	100–180
Average bedtime	<110	<120	100–140
A1C (%)		4.0–6.0%	<7
Preconception			
Before meals		80–110	70–100
2 hours after meals		<155	<140
Pregnancy			
Fasting			60–90
Before meals			60–105
1 hour after meals			100–120
2–6 hours after meals			60–120
2 A.M.–6 A.M.			60–100
A1C (%)			<6
Exception			
Children, elderly, those with hypoglycemia unawareness, and those with frequent severe hypoglycemia			100–200

Putting it all together . . .

So now you have the basics for calculating both types of bolus doses. Sometimes you will need to do just 1 of the calculations, while other situations might require that you use both together. How do you know when to use just 1 or when to use both? As a starting point, keep the following steps in mind.

Pump Bolus Practice

Janet has just started pump therapy, and, working with the members of her diabetes care team, she's developed the following figures for herself:

▍ I:Carb ratio = 1:15
▍ SF = 80
▍ Target BG range is 80–120 mg/dl. She uses 100 mg/dl in her calculations.

Using these numbers, Janet is trying to figure out her bolus dose for lunch on 3 different days. Each day, her lunch contains 65 grams of carbohydrate. She checks her blood glucose before her meal during the 3 days and gets the following readings:

Day 1: BG = 116 mg/dl
Day 2: BG = 231 mg/dl
Day 3: BG = 70 mg/dl

What bolus doses should she use for these 3 days?

Answers:

▍ **Day 1 = 4.3-unit bolus**
Her blood glucose is in her target range, so there's no need for her to use a correction bolus. She simply uses her I:Carb ratio to figure out a food bolus: 65 (the carbs in her lunch) ÷ 15 (the second number of her I:Carb ratio) = 4.3 units

▍ **Day 2 = 5.9-unit bolus**
Her blood glucose is higher than her target, so she needs to add a correction bolus onto her food bolus. Her food bolus is 4.3, the same as it was the day before. Using her SF, she figures out her correction bolus:

(231 [her actual BG] – 100 [her target BG]) ÷ 80 (her SF) = 131 ÷ 80 = 1.6 units
Total bolus = 1.6 units + 4.3 units = 5.9 units

▍ **Day 3 = 3.9-unit bolus**
Her BG is lower than her target BG, so she'll need to subtract a correction bolus from her food bolus. Her food bolus is still 4.3 units. Once again, she'll need to use her SF to calculate a correction bolus.

(70 – 100) ÷ 80 = –30 ÷ 80 = –0.4 units
Total bolus = 4.3 units – 0.4 units = 3.9 units

—OR—

Janet could just eat 15 g of carb to get her blood sugar up to her target range and then simply bolus her food bolus of 4.3 units. If she does this, she needs to be sure not to add the 15 g of carb to her total carb count for the meal. If she does, her food bolus calculation will cover the extra carbs, and she'll just be defeating the purpose.

Extra practice:

Using the same I:Carb ratio, SF, and target BG range as above, figure out Janet's boluses for a meal containing 80 g of carb with the following BG readings:

1. 271 mg/dl
2. 114 mg/dl
3. 62 mg/dl

Answers to extra practice questions:
1. 7.4 units
2. 5.3 units
3. 4.8 units

■ **Step 1:** Try to know how much carbohydrate is in the meal or snack you plan to eat by using nutrition labels and reference books. How many units of insulin are needed to cover this carbohydrate intake?

- If your pre-meal blood glucose is in your target range, you can just use your I:Carb ratio, figure up a food bolus, and move forward with your meal. No extra steps required.
- If your blood glucose is out of range, go to Step 2.

■ **Step 2:** If you're "out of range," how much extra (or less) insulin will you need to "correct" your pre-meal blood glucose? Using your SF, you can quickly determine a correction bolus.

■ **Step 3:** Add (or subtract, depending on what side of your target range you're coming from) the correction bolus with the food bolus, and use this final amount as your total bolus dose. Remember, if you are correcting a low blood sugar, consider treating it with carbohydrate rather than a "negative correction bolus."

Sounds pretty simple, doesn't it? Well, as you move along, you'll find that it's not always this easy. These are just the basic steps you take to determine bolus doses. Sometimes these basics will work perfectly; other times they'll provide frustratingly inconsistent results. Furthermore, as you start your pump therapy, you'll find that your beginning I:Carb ratio and SF aren't perfect. They will need to be evaluated and adjusted to get good control, which we'll discuss below.

But before we move on, you need to be well versed in the basics. Try calculating the examples in the box on page 50 to make sure you're up to speed.

Evaluating and Adjusting Your Bolus Doses

Just like basal rates, your initial bolus doses will need to be evaluated and adjusted. These initial rates are based on estimations and educated guesses; they are the springboards for good, tight therapy. As you move forward, you'll want to ask yourself certain questions about your bolus doses. Does your I:Carb ratio properly cover the carbohydrates you eat? Does your SF accurately correct out-of-range blood glucose readings?

Fortunately, there are ways to answer these questions and evaluate your bolus doses, leading to accurate I:Carb ratios and an on-the-money SF.

As you may remember, the most important step you need to take when evaluating basal rates is to eliminate the variables that affect your basal rate (food, boluses, etc.). The same thing is true for bolus doses. To accurately evaluate your bolus doses, you need to isolate the effects of the bolus. Clearly, the variables that have the most affect on your bolus doses are your basal rates. Before you think about evaluating your bolus doses, your basal rates need to be solid. There will be times when your physician and/or diabetes educator will advise you to change your bolus dose formulas while you're still evaluating your basal rates. However, there's a good chance that once your basal rates are fine-tuned, these bolus changes will be changed once again.

> **First Things First!**
>
> First, evaluate and fine-tune your basal insulin rates.
>
> Then, evaluate and fine-tune your bolus dose formulas.

There are other factors that will affect your bolus doses during an evaluation, as well. It's best not to evaluate bolus doses on days when:

- You are under stress
- You have had alcohol
- You have exercised or have been very active
- You are ill or not feeling well
- You've had frequent low blood sugar reactions

Evaluating your insulin-to-carbohydrate ratio

If your blood glucose consistently returns to your target range about 4 hours after your meals, you can be confident that your I:Carb is working like it should. If not, then you need to spend some time evaluating and adjusting your I:Carb ratio.

An I:Carb evaluation needs to take place when you check your blood glucose before a meal and find that it's right in your target range. If you need to use a correction bolus to get your level down, it won't be the best time to evaluate your I:Carb, because its effects will not be isolated. Once you've found your blood glucose levels are on track, you can begin the evaluation.

With your glucose levels in range, your first step is to simply calculate your food bolus, take the bolus, and then eat. However, not every meal is ideal for an evaluation. Primarily, you need to be able to accurately estimate the carbohydrate content; after all, you're trying to figure out if the insulin you take per gram of carbohydrate is working correctly. You also need to choose a meal that's low in fat, say no more than 10 grams. Fat can affect your sensitivity to insulin and delay the emptying of your stomach (see Chapter 11 for more about dietary fat's effects on insulin sensitivity).

After you eat, monitor your blood glucose every hour or 2 for the next 4 hours. Two hours after eating, you should expect your blood glucose to be *higher* than your pre-meal glucose since your food bolus is still at work. It's perfectly normal to see an increase of about 40–80 mg/dl. After 4 hours, your blood glucose should be at, or very close to, your target range (Fig. 5-2).

If your blood glucose is above target after your evaluation, then you obviously need more insulin for your carbohydrate. In other words, your I:Carb ratio would need to be decreased. For example, if you're using a ratio of 1:15, moving to a ratio of 1:12 would mean you need to bolus more insulin (instead of covering 15 grams of carb, 1 unit of insulin would aim to cover 12). If your blood glucose ends up low, the reverse is true; you're using too much insulin, and you'll need to raise your ratio.

Keep in mind that you're looking for trends in your therapy. One result doesn't necessarily indicate success or failure. That's why it's important to run multiple evaluations at different times in the day before deciding to make any changes. Once you make changes, run more evaluations to see if these changes are effective. Remember to always discuss your results with your physician and/or educator before making any changes.

Sensitivity Factor

The goal of your SF (and the correction bolus it determines) is to return your glucose levels to normal if they are high (if they are low, the "correction" bolus is actually just an amount subtracted from your food bolus). A correction bolus should get your levels to target in about 3–5 hours, depending on the type of insulin you're using (see Chapter 10 for more on insulin profiles).

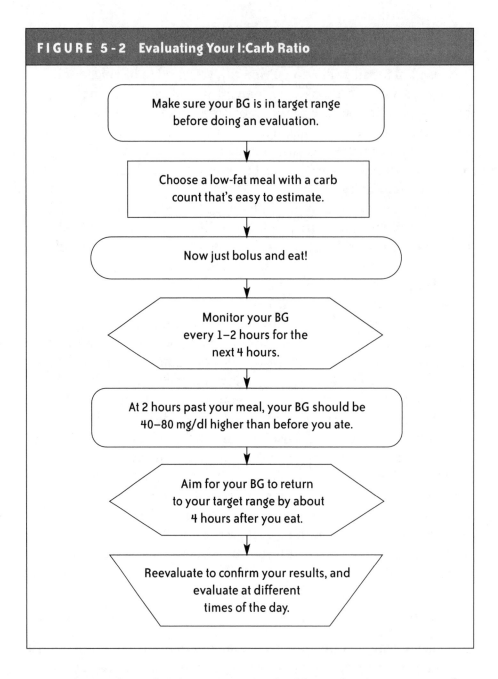

FIGURE 5-2   Evaluating Your I:Carb Ratio

Make sure your BG is in target range before doing an evaluation.

Choose a low-fat meal with a carb count that's easy to estimate.

Now just bolus and eat!

Monitor your BG every 1–2 hours for the next 4 hours.

At 2 hours past your meal, your BG should be 40–80 mg/dl higher than before you ate.

Aim for your BG to return to your target range by about 4 hours after you eat.

Reevaluate to confirm your results, and evaluate at different times of the day.

Fortunately, evaluating your SF is a lot like evaluating your I:Carb ratio, with a couple of changes. First of all, your glucose levels need to be above target, thus requiring a correction bolus. Second, you should not have eaten at least 3 hours or so before you evaluate and should plan to not eat for 4 hours after you bolus. In other words, you need at least a

---

Evaluating Your Sensitivity Factor

▌ To isolate the effects of your SF, begin the evaluation well after your last bolus or food. This means at least 3 hours after a bolus with Humalog/ Novolog or at least 4 hours after a bolus with regular.

▌ If you've met the above time require- ments, take a correction bolus when your blood glucose is high (at least 180 mg/dl) using your SF.

▌ Be sure to check your BG after 2 hours and then again after 4 hours. Make sure you don't eat during this time.

Aim to be within your target range about 4 hours after you bolus.

▌ Rule out other conditions that may be affecting your blood glucose.

▌ Remember to keep detailed records! Actually, if you've been doing frequent blood glucose checks and keeping good records all along, just a thorough review of your logs can give you an indication of how your correction boluses have been working. Look for correction boluses you took when you didn't eat 3 hours before the bolus and 4 hours after; then analyze the results.

7-hour window with no food or additional boluses. Once these criteria have been met, simply take a correction bolus and monitor your blood glucose every hour for the next 4 hours. Keep detailed records that you can show your physician and/or diabetes educator.

Is your SF working? If your blood glucose is within 30 mg/dl of your target blood glucose (the number you used in your bolus calcula- tion), then your SF is right on track. If it's higher than 30 mg/dl above your target, your SF needs to be decreased. Talk to your diabetes care team for help on what you should do.

Timing of correction boluses

The timing of correction boluses can be very important and should always be considered. For example, if your blood glucose before you eat is high, your blood glucose after your meal will tend to be better if you're able to take a correction bolus and then wait a bit before eating. On the other hand, if your blood glucose is on the low side, you should prob- ably wait until after you've started eating to bolus your food bolus—or even take it after your meal. You could also try using an extended/square wave bolus over a 30-minute period to cover the meal. This will delay your insulin a bit while your blood glucose increases.

A Final Comment

So now we've covered the basics of the bolus dose. We've talked about everything from estimating an initial I:Carb ratio and SF and using these to figure out bolus doses, to evaluating these numbers and adjusting them to fit your needs. It may seem like a lot of information all at once, and it is. But don't worry; with the help of your diabetes care team and a little extra work, it will all start to make sense. Most importantly, remember that this is not an exact science. Your results won't always be the same. Later in the book, we'll talk more about how to tighten your control by using a different I:Carb ratio and SF for different times of the day and different situations.

Be patient, be diligent, and pay attention, and pretty soon it will all be second nature to you.

6 Carbohydrate Counting and the Pump

If you've had diabetes for a long time, you're probably painfully familiar with the old regimen and restrictions that made-up the "diabetic diet" of the past. Few food choices, absolutely no sugar, specific time frames—altogether a pretty dreary meal plan. Even worse was the guilt and feelings of cheating that came with any occasional splurge. And many doctors did little to discourage these feelings.

Fortunately, as we discussed earlier in the book, a lot has changed in diabetes therapy, including approaches to diet and meal plans. New therapies, such as the pump, allow people with diabetes to more accurately mimic a fully functioning pancreas. This, along with an increased understanding of nutrition, translates into greater freedom for people with diabetes, especially in terms of food.

Perhaps the biggest step forward in our understanding of diabetes nutrition was the discovery that all carbohydrates act pretty much the same way in the body (there are, however, some differences, which we'll soon talk about). Furthermore, of the type of nutrients we regularly consume, carbohydrates have the biggest impact on our blood glucose. Thus, learning how to count the carbohydrates we ingest so that we can accurately "cover" them with our insulin doses is an essential aspect to good diabetes management.

Carbohydrates

Here are some facts about carbohydrates that you may find useful.

- Carbohydrate is your body's main source of energy.
- Most of the carb you eat is converted to glucose, which your body uses as fuel.
- There are 3 main types of carbohydrate:

    - Starch   • Fiber   • Sugar

- Since your body does not break down fiber, it should not be counted as a significant source of carb. In fact, if you eat over 5 grams of fiber with a meal, you can subtract the amount of fiber from your total carb count. For example, if you eat 30 grams of carbohydrate, but 11 grams of fiber, then your total carb count is only 19 grams.
- Most of the time, any food that "grows from the ground" is going to have carbohydrate. However, dairy products and legumes (beans) also have carbohydrate and must be counted in your total carb count.

Foods with Carbohydrate	
Bread, cereal, pasta, and grains	Fruit and fruit juice
Rice and beans	Milk and yogurt
Vegetables, particularly starchy vegetables, such as potatoes, winter squash, corn, and peas	Sugary foods—dessert foods, honey, syrup, soda pop, etc.

Carbohydrates and the Exchange System

If you're familiar with the "old school" of diabetes management, you're probably familiar with the exchange system. You probably also let out a long groan when you read the title of this section. In an attempt to simplify healthy meal planning for people with diabetes, the exchange system inadvertently created a rigid, standardized approach to eating that didn't leave much freedom for the individual. Ultimately, the exchange system hasn't exactly been the most loved method of meal planning.

Then again, the exchange system isn't completely bad. By grouping foods into similar categories of nutritional content and serving size, they simplified healthy eating immensely. In fact, most weight loss systems on the market today employ a similar method of food exchanges.

Food exchanges basically work as follows: Meals are created by combining serving amounts of different foods from specified food lists (i.e., 2 servings bread/starch, 3 servings vegetable, etc.). These food lists contain measured amounts of food similar in nutritional value and calories. Items on these lists are interchangeable; contain similar amounts of carb, protein, and fat; and have a similar impact on your blood glucose. In other words, they can all be exchanged for one another. For example, on the bread/starch list, each serving contains about 15 grams of carb. So, 1/2 cup of mashed potatoes, 1/2 English muffin, 1/3 cup of lentils, or 8 animal crackers would all constitute one serving, since they each have about 15 grams of carb. If your meal called for 1 bread/starch serving, you could choose any of the above to meet this requirement.

Ideally, the exchange system wouldn't be such a bad deal. Unfortunately, this is not an ideal world. For example, if you want more or less servings of a food than your exchange meal calls for, you're out of luck. Furthermore, exchange food lists are standardized. So if you're not in the mood for any of the foods on the list, you're pretty much forced to eat foods you don't want or suffer high or low blood glucose.

Exchange lists vs. carb counting

In 1995, the exchange lists underwent a major reorganization. The primary change was that all the exchange lists were simplified into 3 main groups—carbohydrate, meat, and fat. Foods in the carbohydrate group include starch, fruit, milk, other carbohydrates (snack/dessert foods), and vegetables. One serving of each of these 5 groups contained about 15 grams of carbohydrate, except for vegetables, which required 3 servings to meet the 15-gram criteria.

In addition, all of the exchanges were converted into carbohydrate grams so that people using the exchange system could count the carb content of their meals. The conversion went as shown in Table 6-1.

TABLE 6-1 Amount of Carb in Exchange Servings	
Exchange system approach using the 6 food groups	**Carbohydrate counting**
1 starch	15 g of carb
1 fruit	15 g of carb
1 milk	15 g of carb
1 vegetable	5 g of carb
1 meat	0 g of carb
1 fat	0 g of carb

While this conversion simplified the process, it proved to be less accurate than carb counting using Nutrition Facts labels and reference books. If you're looking to nail down your carbohydrate content exactly, these "rounded" numbers aren't good enough. As a result, matching your insulin to your carb content won't be as precise.

Exchanges or carb counting?

The insulin bolus you take to cover your meal depends on your accuracy in counting the carb content of what you eat. The carb content of the Thanksgiving meal shown in Table 6-2 was counted using two methods:

Table 6-2 Two Methods		
Food Eaten At Meal	**Number of Exchanges and Carb Grams**	**Actual Grams of Carb**
1 (5 1/2 oz) baked potato	2 choices—30 g of carb	34 g of carb
1 1/2 cups sliced carrots	1 choice—15 g of carb	24 g of carb
4 oz roasted turkey	0	0
1/4 cup cranberry sauce	1 1/2 choices—22 g of carb	27 g of carb
1 (8 oz) apple	2 choices—30 g of carb	34 g of carb
8 oz skim milk	1 choice—15 g of carb	12 g of carb
Total	**7 1/2 choices—112 grams of carb**	**131 grams of carb**

the exchange system, and carb counting using weights, measures, and a carb reference book.

Quite a difference! Now let's assume you use an I:Carb ratio of 1:15 at this meal. If you calculated your bolus using the exchange system, your dose would be:

$$112 \text{ g carb} \div 15 = 7.5\text{-unit bolus dose}$$

If you calculated your bolus dose using the more precise carb counting method, your dose would be:

$$131 \text{ g carb} \div 15 = 8.7\text{-unit bolus dose}$$

That's a 1.2-unit difference in the bolus doses, which can lead to higher blood glucoses down the line. (If you're still wondering why carb counting is important, just imagine how far off a guess or estimate would have been!) So, for more accurate bolus dosing, take advantage of food labels, measuring equipment, and carb reference books to accurately measure your carb intake. It may take a little extra work, but the added attention is worth it.

Counting Your Carbohydrates

Learning to count the carbohydrates in the food you eat requires a number of skills. From reading food labels, to using weights and measurements, to referencing your meals with nutrition facts books—it's an all-encompassing task. If the processes and methods explained in this chapter seem daunting, remember that this is a learning experience. It will become easier with practice.

It might also seem like carb counting takes the joy and pleasure of eating and reduces it to weights and measurements and numbers in

---

Carb Counting Checklist

The following items are essential to effective carbohydrate counting. Make sure you have everything on this checklist as you begin counting carbs.

▌ Measuring cups and spoons

▌ Food scale
▌ Food labels
▌ Carbohydrate counting reference books
▌ Calculator
▌ Patience!

books. Admittedly, this is not that far from the truth in the beginning. However, as you become accustomed to carb counting, you'll develop a feel for the process, an instinct for size and portion, and a knack for assessing how much carbohydrate there is in a meal. It may seem intense at first, but like most things involved with pump therapy, the benefits will far outweigh the burden.

Nutrition Facts Labels in 4 Easy Steps

Nutrition Facts

Serving Size 1/2 cup (114g)
Servings Per Container 4

Amount per Serving

Calories 90   **Calories from Fat** 30

	% Daily Value*
Total Fat 3g	5%
Saturated Fat 0g	0%
Cholesterol 0mg	0%
Sodium 300mg	13%
Total Carbohydrate 13g	4%
Dietary Fiber 3g	12%
Sugars 3g	
Protein 3g	

Vitamin A 80%	•	Vitamin C 60%
Calcium 4%	•	Iron 4%

*Percent Daily Values are based on a 2,000 calorie diet. Your daily values may be higher or lower depending on your calorie needs:

		Calories:	2,000	2,500
Total Fat	Less than		65g	80g
Sat Fat	Less than		20g	25g
Cholesterol	Less than		300mg	300mg
Sodium	Less than		2,400mg	2,400mg
Total Carbohydrate			300g	375g
Dietary Fiber			25g	30g

Calories per gram:
Fat 9 • Carbohydrate 4 • Protein 4

The standardization of Nutrition Facts labels on all food sold in the U.S. is one of the best things to ever happen to people counting their carbs. These labels present all the nutrient information you need to know to keep track of what you eat, but only if you use it correctly. Simply looking at numbers on labels doesn't necessarily translate into helpful nutrition information.

So, you might be asking, "How do I use the Nutrition Facts labels to my advantage?" Hopefully, the following 4 guidelines should help you interpret the information they present.

1. Check the Serving Size

Always start at the top of the label so you won't miss the most important, and the most often overlooked, information on the label—the Serving Size. Most of the time, the serving size listed on the label is quite a bit smaller than the serving you'll actually eat (though it doesn't have to be!). Instead of thinking that the serving size is *telling* you how much you *should* eat, use it as a guide to accurately measure the carb and fat that you'll *actually* eat. For example, if the serving size indicates a 1/2 cup as a serving, and you'll probably actually eat 1 cup, you should double the amount of carb and fat listed on the label.

2. Check the Fat

As you work your way down the label, you'll notice the Total Fat. This category will tell you immediately if this particular food is a good "heart healthy" choice. In this case, there are only 3 grams of fat, which is generally considered low fat and heart healthy. In addition, none of the fat is saturated fat, so that's even better!

Another thing you should consider is the amount of calories coming from fat. Right above the Total Fat listing, directly across from the Calories, is the Calories from Fat listing. Generally, you want less than half of your calories to come from fat. In this case, 30 of the 90 calories in a serving come from fat, or about 1/3, which is a pretty good ratio.

3. Check the Total Carbohydrate

This category, as you can imagine, contains the most relevant information for carb counting. All types of carbs are included in this number (starch, fiber, and sugar). In the example above, you can see that 1 serving contains 13 grams of carbohydrate. This would be the number you would use in your bolus calculations (depending on your fiber content, which we'll get to in just a second). Remember, if you eat 1 cup, or 2 servings, you'll need to double the amount of carbs listed to 26.

Important Note: Occasionally, people will confuse the total weight of the serving (listed next to Serving Size) with the amount of carbohydrate since both are listed in grams. Be sure you do not make this mistake. This could drastically affect your bolus dose calculations.

4. Check the Dietary Fiber

Dietary Fiber is listed right below the Total Carbohydrate. Since fiber is a carbohydrate, it is counted in the Total Carbohydrate (in this case, making up 3 of the 13 grams). However, your body does not digest fiber, so it will not be converted to calories or have an impact on your blood glucose. When you first begin pump therapy, subtract the fiber grams from

Focus on Food Labels	
1. Read the "Nutrition Facts" on the food label	5. Add up the grams of carb in your serving
2. Find the serving size	6. Adjust for fiber
3. Compare your serving…weigh and measure what you plan to eat	7. (Optional) Compare total grams of carbohydrate and fat with reference foods to better determine the impact on blood glucose
4. Look for the grams of total carbohydrate and total fat	

your total carbohydrate count for your bolus calculations. As you move along with your therapy, you'll notice that different forms of carbohydrate affect your blood glucose differently. At this point, you may want to subtract the fiber only when the fiber content is 5 grams or more. Now you can see the benefits of high-fiber foods. After deducting the fiber, a 1/2 cup serving now only has 10 grams of carb!

Measuring Accurate Portions

Without a doubt, carbohydrate counting is only as accurate as the portions you measure. You can consult reference books and nutrition labels all you want, but if what you're *actually* eating is different from what you *thought* you were eating, you'll have no idea how many carbs are being converted to blood glucose in your body. If you want tight control, measuring your portions is the key.

Accurately measuring your food, however, is no easy feat. It will take practice and experience to get where you need to be. The following tips will help you get started.

■ Your first step is to become more familiar with what typical portions look like on your plate. For example, is that 1 cup of pasta on your plate, or is it really 1 1/2 cups of pasta? The difference, while hard to notice visually, can make a big difference in your insulin requirements (57 grams of carb requires quite a bit more insulin than 38 grams). This is why measuring is important at first. As you become more familiar with the amount that you typically eat, you won't need to weigh and measure your foods as often.

■ Portion sizes tend to increase over time! If you notice that your blood glucose levels are rising more than usual after meals, go back to the weights and measurements to keep yourself on track.

■ Different foods need to be measured differently. Some foods work best measured by *volume*, while others are better measured by *weight*. Some foods may include a little of both.

■ Cereal, pasta, and rice can be measured in "nested" measuring cups. Be sure to use a knife to level the top.

■ Make sure to pay attention to where you're getting your information and how the measurements are made…does your reference book state the servings as raw or cooked? There's a big difference.

■ Beverages and liquid foods can be measured with a graduated measuring cup. Put the cup on a level surface and look at it at eye level.

■ Bread products can be weighed on a food scale. In general, 1 oz usually contains about 15 grams of carb. However, there are lots of different breads, so this may not always be the case. Furthermore, some "bread" products, such as muffins and dessert breads, will have a lot of added fat and carbohydrate.

■ Using a carb reference book, fruits can also be weighed on a scale.

■ When using a measuring spoon to measure foods such as jam, jelly, and peanut butter, be sure to level the top with a knife.

Measuring Comparisons for the Real World		
Starch	Pasta and rice 1/2 cup 1 cup 1 medium potato	 The size of your palm The size of your fist The size of a computer mouse
Fruit	1 small piece of fresh fruit 1/2 cup canned fruit 1 bunch of grapes	The size of a tennis ball The size of a baseball The size of a light bulb
Milk	8 oz, or 1 cup	The size of a small coffee cup
Vegetables	1 1/2 cups cooked, or 3 cups raw	The size of 3 lightbulbs

> **Remember!**
>
> **Precise measurements equal precise insulin doses! Even small errors can affect your carb counting efforts, especially with a meal containing several different foods.**

Different carbs, different results

Not all carbs react the same way in your body. Studies have shown that sugar is no longer a "no-no," that carbs are just carbs, and they should all be treated the same way. Well, that's not always true. People with diabetes *can* fit sugar into their diet, but that doesn't mean that a piece of bread and a lollipop will have the same effect on your blood sugar.

As you look to tighten your control, you may become aware that different types of carbohydrates can have different effects on your blood glucose. Learning about the *glycemic index*, a list of foods organized according to their ability to raise your blood glucose, may be helpful. Most importantly, you'll need to keep detailed records of how certain types of foods raise your blood glucose as opposed to others. We'll discuss this in more in depth in Chapter 11, when we talk about nutrition and its relation to pump therapy. For now, keep in mind that not all carbs are created equally and that if you notice irregularities in your readings where you think there should be none, this might be the source.

But all of this is getting a little advanced. As you start pump therapy and carb counting, your main objective is to accurately measure your portions and carbohydrate content. The details will come later.

One last thing

Your focus on counting carbs doesn't mean you can forget everything you know about eating healthy. Just because you're counting carbs doesn't mean you shouldn't also be paying attention to other nutrients, such as protein and fat. Carbohydrate may have the biggest impact on your blood sugar, but it's not the only nutrient that has an impact on your body as a whole. In fact, large amounts of fat and protein *can* affect your blood glucose by delaying the emptying of your stomach and slowing down your absorption of carbs. Further, high-fat meals will reduce your sensitivity (responsiveness) to insulin, resulting in after-meal high blood glucose.

Remember—carbs are important, but they're not the only things you eat. Paying attention to all your nutrients will give you tighter control and better health down the road.

For more information

Check the resource section on page 175 for carbohydrate reference books that can help you determine the carb content of the foods you eat. Be sure to pay close attention to the abbreviations at the top of the pages in reference books. Mistaking carbohydrate listings for calorie listings can have disastrous results!

7 Wearing the Pump

Pump therapy is more than simply calculating doses to cover your insulin requirements. It is more than boluses, basal rates, and carb counting. Pump therapy requires that you wear a device that will be connected to your body day and night. Along with practical issues, such as learning to properly insert the catheter or cannula (needle) and wear the pump comfortably and safely, it can sometimes take a while getting used to having an outward sign of diabetes. In this chapter, we'll offer some guidance about infusion sets, some pointers about wearing the pump, and some tips to help you introduce your pump to other people in your life.

Deciding About Infusion Sets

A lot of people starting out on the pump don't realize that problems with infusion catheters are the number 1 cause of unexplained high blood glucose. Using the right type of catheter and skin tape can greatly reduce this risk. So which type of infusion set is right for you? Before we can answer this question, we should make some comments on infusion sets in general.

There are two type of infusion sets—metal and teflon (plastic). Metal sets have the advantage of not kinking, so there's less risk of insulin non-delivery. However, these sets can't be disconnected from the pump (which can be inconvenient for bathing, exercise, or intimacy) and are more easily felt than the plastic sets, especially with bending or activity. All of the pump companies offer infusion sets that either insert "straight" (at a 90-degree angle) or obliquely (at a 30- to 45-degree angle). Most infusion sets come with an *insertion device*, although some can only be inserted manually.

The following gives a brief rundown of some of the sets available and what to expect from each:

- Catheters that pass directly into the skin at a 90-degree angle (such as the Medtronic MiniMed Sof-set and Disetronic Ultraflex) are popular, but these catheters are more prone to kink. With thin individuals or children, kinking can occur because the catheter tip is pressing against the muscle layer underlying the subcutaneous fat—changing to an infusion set that has a shorter, 6-mm–long cannula can help with this problem. Kinking can also occur if the catheter tubing is inadvertently pulled, and usually happens during the summer when heat and perspiration loosen the tape that holds the set. If the catheter kinks, your insulin can't be delivered and your glucose levels are going to shoot up. If you use a Sof-set or Ultraflex catheter, get into the habit of examining your catheter after you remove it. If you notice kinking, you might consider changing to a Silhouette/Tender/Comfort catheter.
- The Silhouette/Tender/Comfort catheter passes through the skin obliquely (at an angle) and is much less prone to kinking. Oblique catheters are also particularly helpful for thin individuals who don't have much subcutaneous fat. Remember, if you insert this catheter in your abdomen, you have to position it horizontally (from side-to-side). If you position it vertically (up and down), it can kink when you bend forward. Using an insertion device with these catheters can sometimes cause bruising and can lead to erratic insulin absorption.
- If you use the Medtronic MiniMed Quick-set catheter, be careful not to grip the base attached to the skin when you detach the tubing—this can dislodge the catheter and disrupt insulin delivery.

Keeping all of this in mind can be a little confusing. There's a lot to consider when deciding on an infusion set. Talk with your diabetes care team. They can show you a variety of different infusion sets and help you decide which one is right for you.

Deciding About Infusion Sites

As you decide about where to insert your catheter, keep the following in mind:

- The best area to place your catheter is on your abdomen. Insulin is absorbed faster and more predictably in your abdomen than anywhere else in your body.
- Even though the abdomen is your best option, using the same spot over and over again can thicken your skin, which interferes with absorption of insulin. Other sites to try include the upper part of your outer thighs or the back of your hips.
- Avoid areas of your body that might be constricted (such as your belt line) or bumped (such as the seat of your pants).
- Painful insertion can indicate that you've inserted too close to muscle tissue.

Finding the right infusion site can take some trial and error. It may take a few insertions before you find the sites that work best for you and your lifestyle. Remember, comfort is an important factor in deciding where you want your infusion site. If you're not comfortable, you're not going to be happy with the pump.

Worthwhile Habits

- Check your infusion site daily to make sure that the set is secure and there is no evidence of infection (see page 71 for more on signs of infection).
- Change your infusion site every 2–3 days as recommended by your diabetes care team. This will reduce the risk of infection. Changing and rotating your sites often can prevent thickening under your skin.
- Clean the insertion site carefully with an antiseptic solution (such as Hibiclens or Betadine). Wipe and allow it to dry before inserting the infusion set. You can also use an antibacterial soap (such as Dial or Hibiclens) in the shower.
- Check your tubing daily for air bubbles.

Smart Pumping Tip

When in doubt, change it out!
If you have unexplained blood glucose levels of 250 mg/dl or greater
2 times in a row, change the cartridge and infusion set and check for
ketones. Take fast-acting insulin by syringe as directed by your health care
professional.

- Rotate your sites at each set-change to prevent overuse of one area and a resulting thickening of the skin. Move your new site at least 1 inch away from your old site and 1 inch away from your navel, scars, and any hardened tissue.
- Choose a site that you can easily see. This will be helpful if you need to troubleshoot any potential catheter problems.
- Change your set early in the day. This will give you a chance to see if your insulin is infusing properly through the catheter. If your insulin is not infusing correctly, your blood glucose results will be higher than usual.
- Always check your blood glucose 1–2 hours after inserting a new infusion set.
- Always keep an extra infusion set with you at all times. Call for new infusion sets when you open your last box!

Checking for Infection

Catching the early signs of infusion site infection is the key to ensuring that the problem doesn't get out of hand. Look for the following signs of an initial infection:

- Discomfort or tenderness
- Redness and inflammation
- Warmth, discharge, or drainage

If you notice any of these features *and* also have a fever, immediately change your infusion set and contact your health care provider. If you notice these symptoms but *do not* have a fever, immediately change the infusion site and apply a topical, antibacterial ointment. If the symp-

> **Caution!**
>
> Contact your health care provider immediately if you have a firm lump under your skin at a catheter site—this could be an abscess.

toms don't get any better within 24 hours, get in touch with your health care provider.

If you notice a lump under your skin at a catheter site, get in touch with your health care provider immediately. This could be an abscess, which could mean serious trouble.

Tips for other site problems

- If you develop irritation at the catheter site, you may have a mild allergy. Or, there might be some friction from the tape you're using. If it's the tape, *barrier agents* may be helpful. Tegaderm, TegadermHP, or Polyskin are helpful dressings, and Skin-Prep is an effective "wipe-on" barrier. These products provide a base for the clear covering. The catheter is inserted through the barrier, and then the clear covering is applied on top of the catheter.
- If you have extremely sensitive skin, removing tape can cause irritation. Tape removers, such as Detachol and Uni-Solve, dissolve the tape and the adhesive, reducing damage to your skin.
- Sometimes perspiration may cause tape to lose its stickiness. If you have this problem, try wiping the site with an adhering agent such as IV Prep, Skin-Prep, or Skin Tac H, and allow it dry before inserting your set. Applying an unscented antiperspirant to the skin *around* (not on) the insertion site before you insert your infusion set can also help.
- If you have frequent infections at your catheter site, you might want to use a stronger antiseptic to prepare the site and minimize the ways germs and bacteria can come in contact with the infusion area. Always be sure to wash your hands thoroughly before you insert the catheter, and never "blow" on the site to dry it.
- To lower discomfort from inserting the catheter, try pre-treating the site with an anesthetic cream, such as EMLA.

Smart Pumping Tip

The problem:
High blood glucose after changing your infusion set.

Things to consider:

| Are you forgetting to fill the new cannula with insulin after inserting a new set?** Forgetting this step may result in you not getting insulin delivery for several hours. For example, if your basal rate is 0.5 units/hour, and the set you use has a cannula that holds 1 unit of insulin, you won't be getting any basal insulin for 2 hours if you forget to fill your cannula. Check with your diabetes care team or your infusion set instructions for the amount of insulin required to fill your cannula.

| Did you bolus shortly *before* changing your set?** Some pump users have noticed insulin leaking out of their infusion site if they "pull a site" within an hour or so of delivering a bolus. The insulin from a bolus actually pools under the skin until it is all absorbed. If you remove the infusion set from the site soon after a bolus, you may not get all of the insulin you bolused. If you think this is the case, try to either change your set before a meal or bolus, or keep your old set in for an hour or 2 after you bolus (even if you've inserted a new set somewhere else).

| Where is your pump in relation to your infusion site when you connect the tube or inject your set?** When you have finished priming your set, you should notice a drop of insulin at the end of the tube (or needle). However, if you are standing and have the pump lower than your site, the insulin will suck back into the tubing before you connect (or insert the needle). To prevent this, hold your pump higher than the infusion site when you first go to connect or inject the needle. Some people hold the pump under their chin, clip it onto their collar, or simply sit down so the pump is higher than the site—and gravity is working with you. This will prevent the insulin from sucking back into the tubing.

For more information on troubleshooting unexplained high blood glucose readings, see Chapter 9.

■ Pump companies have a wealth of information and advice when it comes to infusion site problems. Contacting them with problems might be worthwhile.

Pump Wearing FAQs

A big worry of most new pump users is where, when, and how to conveniently and comfortably wear their new pump. The good news is you can wear the pump just about anywhere! You'll be surprised at how creative you can be. However, different situations call for different pump-wearing solutions. The following questions probably sound familiar. Hopefully, they'll be helpful in answering your where-does-this-go concerns.

Where do I wear this thing?

First of all, count your lucky stars you've got over 20 years of pump technology to work with. When the first pumps were introduced, they were the size of a large backpack, awkward, and extremely heavy. Imagine having to walk around with that sack of potatoes on your back all day.

Today, insulin pumps are so small they're often mistaken for beepers or cell phones. As you can imagine, this makes modern pumps much easier to wear. Most pump users clip their pump to their waistband or belt, or simply slip it in their pocket. Of course, if you're a woman, you may not always have a waistband or pocket. If not, you can wear your pump in your bra (you'll want to slip the pump into a baby sock to prevent sticking or irritation) or inside your pantyhose next to your stomach. You may even want to design your own "pocket" to attach to the inside of a special garment (like a wedding dress or evening gown). Your pump company will also have a large assortment of accessories designed to make wearing the pump easier and more comfortable.

What do I do with the pump when I'm exercising or playing sports?

All of the pump companies offer a sturdy, heavy-duty "sport case" for your pump. These sport cases come in all shapes and sizes, ranging from a semi-soft, flexible material to a solid, impact-resistant case. Some can be water-resistant or waterproof and most can be worn around your waist or in a harness on your back.

For contact sports and prolonged activities where wearing the pump wouldn't be convenient, you might consider taking an injection of Lantus (glargine) to provide some basal insulin. See Chapter 14 for more on this alternative approach.

What do I do with my pump when I shower?

If your pump is water-resistant, you can wear it in the shower in a specially designed plastic shower pouch. However, most pump users temporarily remove their pump while they shower because it can be a little more convenient. If you decide to remove your pump for a short time (less than an hour), you probably won't require any insulin replacement. But be sure to check your blood sugar once you reconnect, and correct for any high blood sugars if they arise.

What do I do if I want to go swimming or spend a day at the beach?

Some pumps are waterproof and can be worn in the water without any problems. However, others are merely water-*resistant* and should not be submerged in water without using a waterproof, impact-resistant case. When dealing with situations that include water, keep the following in mind:

- There are times when you may want to "go off the pump" for an extended pump "vacation." If so, you'll need to know how to safely return to an injection-based insulin regimen made up of a combination of short- and long-acting insulin (see Chapter 14). Check with your diabetes care team before making this move.
- If you plan to spend the day at the beach (1–4 hours or longer), you may want to remove your pump for the day. This will require periodic insulin boluses to replace your basal insulin, to cover any food eaten, and to correct for any high blood glucose. You'll also need to check your blood glucose more frequently. Remember to consider swimming an "activity" and adjust your insulin boluses accordingly.
- If you plan to remove your pump for an hour or less, perhaps for a quick swim, you shouldn't require any insulin replacement. This would be similar to removing your pump for the shower. This will also allow you to keep your pump away from direct sunlight and sand. Just like you did with the shower, make sure you check your blood glucose before reconnecting and use a correction bolus if needed.

Where do I put the pump while I'm sleeping?

This really depends on personal preference and your sleeping patterns. If you (and your partner) tend to sleep calmly, without much tossing and turning, and don't want the pump attached to your sleepwear, you can place the pump next to you on the mattress. If you use long tubing with your infusion set (42 inches or more), you can slip your pump under your pillow or place it in your nightstand. However, if you tend to roll around a lot while you sleep, you'll probably want to find a way to attach the pump to your clothes. Some sleepwear has pockets that you could slip the pump into, or you might be able to fashion a pouch in the leg or waistband of your pajamas.

What if I roll over on my pump, tubing, or infusion set in my sleep?

You'll soon learn that your pump and the infusion sets/tape are extremely durable. Typically, after the first few nights sleeping with the pump, you'll begin to feel more comfortable and trust the sturdiness of your pump and infusion set. Pump buttons require a certain amount of force to be activated, so you're not going to activate them by brushing up against something or accidentally rolling over on them. Further, the tape attaching your tubing is designed to hold for 2–3 days, so unless you're rolling somersaults in your sleep, you should be fine.

What do I do with the pump during times of intimacy?

For those intimate times, infusion sets can be conveniently and temporarily disconnected from the tubing/pump. Remember, do not disconnect the tubing for more than 1 hour or you'll need to use insulin replacement. During these times, it's also recommended that you put your pump in "suspend" mode (stopped) so that the pump will sound an alarm in case you accidentally fall asleep before reconnecting the tubing.

Now That It's There: Introducing the Pump to Others

Once you start wearing the pump, you start wearing a visible sign of your diabetes. For some, this can be a problem; so much of a problem that they choose not to start pump therapy. For others, the effects are less threatening. But no matter what your own views may be, talk of your diabetes is bound to arise more often. Thus, it's helpful to know how to handle these situations and how to introduce the pump to others in your life. How you communicate about your diabetes can have a big impact on how people perceive you and your diabetes.

In the following section, we'll discuss how to talk about your pump with 2 different groups of people. The first is the group of people with whom you have the most contact and from whom you require continuing support—family and friends. The second group is made up of people who may just be curious about your pump and who play no role in your ongoing support. While this may be oversimplifying your social life, for general purposes, you'll find that approaching conversations about your pump with these 2 groups in mind makes the discussion easier.

Communicating about diabetes in general

Before we begin talking specifically about how to approach conversations with either of the groups mentioned above, we should probably talk about how to discuss diabetes in general. When talking about diabetes, keep the following 2 concepts in mind:

- **How you think about diabetes will color how you talk about it.** If you feel ashamed of having diabetes, or feel that any complications you run into with diabetes are entirely your fault, you're going to communicate this "shame-and-blame" to others. If you were always mentioning things like your "bad blood sugars" or calling yourself a "bad diabetic," would you blame others for being reluctant to help?
- **If you talk like you have 100% control over your blood glucose levels, then others will expect this from you.** Anyone who lives with diabetes needs to understand that despite the wonderful recent advances in diabetes therapy (pumps, rapid-acting insulin, etc.), these are not perfect tools and will never provide perfect control of blood sugar levels. And this is something that you need to express to others. For example, if you're always saying things like, "I should have seen that low blood sugar coming," or, "I can't believe I let high blood sugars affect my performance on that test," people will believe that anytime your blood glucose is less than perfect, you're to blame.

Talking with Group 1—family and friends

- **The people who will provide you with ongoing support need the "Big Picture," as well as the nitty-gritty details about pump**

therapy. Start by telling them about the common myths and mistaken ideas about the pump that many people have (even those who know a thing or two about diabetes). In terms of the "Big Picture," it's important that your friends and family know that the pump is not a "smart" machine that automatically regulates your blood sugar while you kick back and sip martinis in a diabetic bliss. The pump is not a cure; it does not act like a human pancreas. The people around you must also understand that pump therapy doesn't mean you can eat anything you want. This is another common misconception. As for the small details, it might be best to make a list of all the daily tasks recommended for pump users, so your friends and family can see what all goes into pump therapy. They should also be aware of the alarms on your pump and what they mean, just in case something goes wrong. Some pump users even like to bring their significant others to pump training sessions, just so they're well versed in pump care. However, this is a personal choice and may not always be practical.

■ **It is critical that you tell each person in your ongoing support group "specifically" how he or she can help**. Perhaps you'd like your partner to learn how to enter bolus doses or learn about infusion sites. Or maybe you don't want anyone but you touching your pump, and you'd just like extra time to check your blood sugars. Maybe you could use some help getting supplies or help remembering to pack everything you need for a trip. Only you know what help you need, and it's important to let the people you're close to know what exactly you would like help with. If you let those around you know that diabetes is not a "do-it-yourself" disease and that there are specific ways you would like their help, this can work to prevent the destructive cycle of "miscarried helping." Miscarried helping occurs when well-meaning help from friends and family members undermines your ability to care for yourself. If you feel blamed or nagged, there's a good chance that your first reaction will be to resist what you're being told to do, just to show that you have control over your life. Let the people around you know that they need to be supportive, not overbearing.

■ **If you experience a serious personal problem with someone because of your pump therapy, ask a member of your diabetes care team for help and advice.** For example, if your boss tells you that you cannot wear a pump in your workplace, ask for help from your health care provider. Perhaps he or she can get in touch with your boss and explain why it's important that you wear the pump at work. Or perhaps a family member feels threatened or scared by the pump, so much so that he or she will not ride in a car with you while you're driving. A health care professional may be able to calm his or her fears, or at the very least, give you a referral to someone who could help. With more and more children taking advantage of pump therapy, problems at school with faculty and classmates are becoming more common as well. You might ask a member of your diabetes care team if he or she wouldn't mind giving a presentation and educating classmates and personnel about pump therapy, although this could be embarrassing for your child. If so, a more low-key approach to educating schoolmates and teachers could also be explored.

Talking with Group 2—coworkers, acquaintances, and everyone else

■ **Be prepared for misunderstanding.** Many people may mistake your pump for a pager or a cell phone. An airport security guard may ask you to remove it before boarding a plane, or an usher at a live performance may ask you to turn it off, not realizing that it's a medical device. In situations like these, it's best to have a brief reply ready—something like, "This looks like a pager, but it's actually a medical device, an insulin pump that helps control my diabetes. I have to wear this to stay healthy. I'm sorry, but I can't remove it or turn it off without seriously risking my health." If you plan on traveling, always carry a letter from your doctor explaining your condition and what supplies you'll need to keep with you while traveling. If you attend a school that doesn't allow pagers or cell phones, provide a written letter from your physician at the beginning of the year to your school administrators and school health professionals. The letter should explain what the pump is and why it is important that you wear it at all times.

■ **Who you tell about the pump is completely up to you.** At some point in your pump therapy, someone you don't know is going to ask, "What is that thing?" How you respond is up to you and your comfort level with the situation. If you want, you can ignore them, or give them a surprised look that indicates what an inappropriate question that is. Or, you can simply say, "This is my insulin pump." Whatever you decide, you are in no way obligated to reveal that you have diabetes or that you're using an insulin pump. Except in certain situations such as the ones mentioned above, who you tell about the pump is *your choice*!

8 Getting a Hold on Physical Activity

If you've been on an insulin regimen for any length of time, you're probably well aware that exercise and activity can have a dramatic effect on your insulin needs. Unfortunately, most people think that "activity and exercise" means hours of strenuous workouts and marathon running. An activity doesn't have to be intense to have an effect on your blood sugar. While it's true that vigorous activity such as running will have a greater effect than, say, washing your car, a lot of everyday activities that you probably take for granted can have an impact on your blood sugar levels.

This chapter will provide you with some basic guidelines for exercising and increasing your basic activity levels while on the pump. We'll discuss how you should adjust your insulin levels and what you eat, as well as practical pointers for infusion site care and pump removal during exercise. We'll talk about how exercise affects your glucose metabolism more in depth in Chapter 12.

Give It a Rest, Speedy

When you first start pump therapy, a member of your diabetes care team will probably suggest that you not exercise while you're still assessing and adjusting your basal rates. Take this advice to heart. During the first few days of your therapy, it's best to eliminate all of the factors that affect your blood glucose levels. And this doesn't just mean 3-hour bike rides; planting a garden in your backyard can have a pretty big impact as well.

However, if you're used to regular exercise and enjoy a regular workout routine, it's best not to keep from exercising *too* long. Not only can an extended break be difficult psychologically, but tuning your basal rates to a non-active lifestyle won't work once you start exercising again. If you have an exercise regimen that you follow closely, talk with your physician or pump trainer about how to work activity into your basal assessment period. While everything may not go as planned, it's best to get you back into your normal routine as soon as possible.

Exercise and Blood Glucose, Food, and Insulin

In general, blood glucose levels tend to drop during exercise. Since your body is working harder than usual and needs more glucose to keep up its heightened pace, you'll need less insulin to keep your blood glucose levels normal. In people without diabetes, the body automatically reduces the level of insulin released during exercise. You, however, must make your own adjustments.

Fortunately, the pump makes adjusting insulin levels for exercise easier. You can either program in a lowered basal rate for exercise, or use less insulin in the food bolus you take with a meal you eat before you exercise. Sometimes you may need to do both. Another option is to eat extra carbohydrate to make up for the increased activity. Which method you choose to use is up to you. We'll talk more later in this chapter about which options are best depending on your situation. You may find that a combination of extra carb and adjusted insulin gives you the results you need.

And if my blood glucose is high?

Sometimes activity can actually raise your blood glucose. This usually happens when your blood sugar is high—and your insulin levels are low—before you start exercising. The increased activity can actually make your blood glucose rise even higher because the low insulin levels trigger your liver to release stored glucose. With little insulin, the glucose can't get into your cells and has nowhere to go. Pretty soon, your body will turn to fat for fuel and ketones will be released into your bloodstream. Now you're at risk for diabetic ketoacidosis. Follow the steps in Table 8-1 if your blood glucose is high before your start exercising.

TABLE 8-1 Exercise and High Blood Glucose	
Type 1	▌ If blood glucose is between 250–300 mg/dl, check for ketones. If ketones are present, **do not** perform physical activity. If ketones are not present, you're okay to exercise. ▌ If blood glucose is 300 mg/dl or higher, check for ketones. If ketones are present, **do not** exercise. If there are no ketones present, go ahead and exercise, but use extreme caution. Perform a second blood glucose reading 10-15 minutes into your physical activity to make sure your glucose level is dropping. If your BG is still rising, stop immediately and take insulin as needed.
Type 2	If you have type 2, you can stay physically active with blood sugars of up to 400 mg/dl. Since your pancreas is still producing insulin, it's very rare for you to be insulin deficient.

Getting Started—Your First Exercise Session

Once you've started making progress with your basal rates and have a general idea about insulin and food adjustments, you can begin to plan your first exercise session with the pump. As you plan your first workout, keep the following in mind:

- Be prepared to monitor your blood glucose at least twice—once at the beginning and once at the end of your session. A midway check would probably be useful as well.
- For your first few sessions, try to exercise at the same time of the day. This will make it easier to measure the exact effect of exer-

Remember!
If you have type 1 diabetes, you should never exercise when ketones are present.

cise on your glucose levels by eliminating other factors. After a few successful workouts, you can move on to other times of the day.

■ Don't plan a full workout right from the start. Keep it small and gradually work your way up. You should keep your first session to about 20-30 minutes. As you move forward, add 5–10 minutes to each session until you get to where you want to be. Moving slowly will allow you to better adapt your pump strategies to your exercise sessions.

■ Don't forget to have food on hand! Even if you've decided to add extra carb to cover your activity, you may need a little something extra just in case you encounter a low blood sugar or you need to stabilize your blood glucose at the end of a session.

So Which Is It—Extra Food? Less Insulin?

Well, that decision is up to you and your diabetes care team. Each strategy has its pros and cons, and it's not always a matter of "either/or." There will be times when you want to use both methods to keep your glucose levels on track. As you weigh your options, keep the following in mind:

■ A lot of people have already used snacking as a way to handle ups and downs when exercising, so they're already comfortable with it. This may or may not be the case for you. If the extra food and calories aren't too much of an issue with you, snacking is usually the easiest way to control your glucose levels as you ease back into an active lifestyle.

■ If you're looking to control your weight, reducing your insulin levels for exercise may be a more effective strategy. It may also be a better option for you if eating before you exercise causes stomach discomfort.

■ Using both strategies is actually pretty common. They work together nicely, and both might be necessary if you plan on engaging in long-term endurance activities.

■ For your first brief exercise periods on the pump, changing basal rates may be a little too complicated. Reducing your bolus doses for your pre-exercise meal or eating some extra carb is usually your best option at first.

■ You may also decide (after discussing this issue with your diabetes care team) that your blood glucose levels don't necessarily put you at risk when you exercise. If this is the case, you may not need to do anything at all.

■ Whatever you decide to do, always be prepared. Make sure you always have your meter, strips, food, and a desire to try to get things right.

Getting Set with Snacking

As we mentioned above, snacking is a popular method for offsetting blood glucose changes during activity. The main goal in snacking is to ensure that the carbs you're eating balance the glucose being used by your muscles to exercise. Too much carb and you're going to have high blood sugars when you're done exercising; too little and you run the risk of hypoglycemia. While there is no single way that works for everyone, there are some guidelines you can follow to get your glucose levels where you want them.

■ If your blood glucose is more than 250 mg/dl, check for ketones. If you have ketones, this means your insulin levels are low and exercise isn't a good idea. If your blood glucose is high, always check for ketones before you exercise.

■ The most common question related to exercise and snacking is, "How much should I eat?" This depends on how your blood glucose responds to activity. As a general rule of thumb, 15–30 grams of carbohydrate will cover somewhere between 30–60 minutes of activity. A sports bar or a light snack should cover you for 45–60 minutes. If you're using a sports drink, juice, or hard candy as your source of carbohydrate, keep extra supplies handy while you're exercising. These types of carbs get used up quickly and will usually only cover about 5–10 minutes of exercise. However, they do provide a quick source of energy and can be very effective if you spread them out during the course of your activity.

■ If your blood glucose is normal and you're about to start a vigorous activity, drink some juice or eat a rapidly absorbed carb snack before you begin. Your muscles tend to zap a lot of glucose in the first 5–10 minutes of exercise. These carbs will cover this dramatic upswing in glucose use.

What to Eat? Snack Options for Exercise				
Product	Calories	Carbohydrate (g)	Protein (g)	Fat (g)
Small apple	60	15	0	0
Peanutbutter Nabs (4)	130	15	3	7
Gatorade (8 oz)	70	17	0	0
Powerade (8 oz)	70	19	0	0
PR Bar	190	19	14	2
Chewy Granola Bar	120	21	2	3
GU (sports gel)	100	25	0	0
Luna	180	25	10	4
Kellogg's Nutra-Grain	140	27	2	3
Snickers Bar	280	35	4	14
PowerBar	230	45	10	2

- You may have a tendency to cover your extra food with a bolus before you exercise. This shouldn't be necessary. In fact, it will probably be counterproductive. Exercise first and then check your blood glucose levels after your workout. If you're still high, then you can bolus and consider exploring different options with your diabetes care team for your next workout. We'll talk more about high blood glucose and exercise later in Chapter 12.
- You may need a snack after your workout, as well. If your blood glucose is less than 100 mg/dl *after* your workout (or less than 120 mg/dl if you have hypoglycemia unawareness), eat a 15- to 30-gram carb snack immediately.

Is it working?

To determine whether or not your exercise snack is working, focus on your blood glucose readings *after* you exercise. Certain signs will tell you whether or not you're getting the results you want.

- Start by setting a post-exercise target range that will put you at the least risk of a low blood sugar reaction. Remember to add a few points as a buffer. A reasonable target range is around 100–140 mg/dl. If you have hypoglycemia unawareness, your target range will need to be a bit higher (for example, 120–160 mg/dl).

Talk with your health care provider to nail down a range that works for you.

■ Check your blood glucose immediately after your activity. If you wait too long, you'll miss your opportunity to take action against low glucose levels.

Caution!

Don't rely on the usual signs and symptoms of a low blood glucose reaction to tip you off while you're exercising. The symptoms of a reaction—sweating, fatigue, shakiness, increased heart rate, inability to concentrate—are also caused by exercising and high activity. So with exercise, it's often hard to sense when your glucose levels are low. In fact, it's possible to exercise right through a reaction and not even know it!

■ Your glucose levels will likely continue to drop after you exercise. In fact, you can experience low blood glucose up to 24–36 hours after strenuous exercise. This means that if your blood glucose reading is 115 mg/dl at the end of a session, and you drop another 30 mg/dl, your final reading is going to be about 85 mg/dl. This is low, but it's manageable. However, if your reading is 85 mg/dl at the end of the session, there's a good chance you're going to drop down into hypoglycemic ranges. Levels this low below your target range directly after exercise probably call for a snack. After strenuous activity, remember to check your blood glucose during the night as well, to make sure you don't suffer a low while you sleep.

■ Never wait to see "if" you're going to suffer a hypoglycemic reaction. If at the end of your workout your glucose levels are running at the bottom end of your target range or below, odds are that you're going to become hypoglycemic. Remember, hypoglycemia is a lot easier to *prevent* than it is to *treat*. So an extra little snack to keep your glucose levels up may be wise.

■ On the other hand, you don't want to overestimate your carb intake. You may not need as much snack as you think. Carefully watching your glucose levels and reacting sensibly is the best way to get into your target range.

Getting Set with Insulin Adjustment

Maybe eating extra carb isn't getting you the results you want. Maybe having extra food on your stomach while you exercise is uncomfortable. Maybe you're looking to control your weight. Maybe you just want tighter control over your glucose levels when you exercise. There are lots of reasons that can lead you to consider adjusting your insulin for exercise. However, before you start adjusting, ask yourself the following questions:

- What time do I plan on exercising?
- Which insulin delivery will be having the most impact on my blood glucose—the basal or bolus?
- How much do I want to adjust my insulin?
- What is a safe glucose range for me at the end of my activity?

Here are some guidelines that should help you with the process:

- In general, exercise sessions lasting longer than 30 minutes will require extra carbohydrate or adjustments to your insulin levels.
- Adjust the insulin that will have the most effect while you exercise, whether it be basal or bolus. Remember that as you first start exercising with the pump, cutting a meal bolus or eating an extra snack is easier than adjusting basal rates.
- Adjustments in your insulin can be different depending on the *type, length,* and *frequency* of your exercise program.

We mentioned above that when adjusting your insulin doses, you need to figure out which type of insulin—basal or bolus—will have the most effect on your activity session. Well, how do you do that? Basically, depending on when you plan to exercise and the type of insulin in your pump, you'll need to determine whether or not your workout will be affected by your bolus dose. If so, you'll want to adjust your bolus dose. If not, you'll want to adjust your basal rate. It's that simple.

Adjusting your bolus

- The first thing you need to do is figure out if your exercise session is going to fall within the time frame of your last bolus. If you use Humalog/Novolog, an exercise session within 2 hours of your last bolus will fall within your bolus time frame. For regular insulin, the cutoff is 4 hours. In either situation, if your workout or period of activity falls within your bolus time frame, your bolus dose should be decreased to account for the activity.

- When decreasing your bolus dose for exercise, go ahead and calculate the dose like you normally would using your Insulin-to-Carbohydrate ratio. In the beginning, take this number and decrease it by 25%. As you move forward with your therapy, this number will be refined to better match your insulin needs during exercise.

- Obviously, how much carbohydrate you eat and how vigorous your activity is will determine how much you need to reduce your bolus. Responses vary from person to person, and it will more than likely take some careful record keeping and experimentation to find out how much you need to adjust your bolus doses for exercise.

TABLE 8-2 If your blood glucose immediately after physical activity is:		
Less than 100 mg/dl (hypoglycemia unawareness <120 mg/dl)	Between 100 and 140 mg/dl (hypoglycemia unawareness = 120–160 mg/dl)	Greater than 140 mg/dl (hypoglycemia unawareness >160 mg/dl)
Snack immediately: 15–30 g of carbohydrate. Increase your snack or decrease your insulin dose for your next physical activity session.	Success! Your insulin/snack adjustment for physical activity is right on target. Revise your adjustments as your physical activity increases.	Increase your insulin dose or decrease your snack for your next physical activity session. Rule out hypoglycemia during activity as a possible cause—check your blood glucose level during your next physical activity session.

Remember!
For your first few exercise sessions with the pump, it's usually easiest to adjust a bolus dose or use snacks to control your glucose levels during exercise or activity, as opposed to adjusting your basal rate.

Adjusting your basal insulin

- If it looks like your exercise session isn't going to fall within your peak bolus time frame and you have decided against snacking, you'll probably want to set a *temporary basal rate*. For exercise, you may want to set a rate that's about 10–50% lower than your normal basal rate for that period of time. Once again, the higher the activity, the lower your rate needs to be set. Activities such as brisk walking, tennis, or golf will sometimes need as much as a 50% reduction.

- When you program how long your temporary rate will last, be sure that it not only covers your exercise session, but covers a period of time after your session as well. After exercise, your muscles will still be taking up glucose from your blood to replenish the glucose stores that were used up during exercise. Going back to your normal basal rate immediately after an exercise session can cause your blood glucose to drop rapidly.

Temporary Basal Rates and Activity

Different types of activities call for different adjustments to your basal rates. Generally, the more strenuous the exercise or activity, the bigger the adjustment to the basal rate. For example, Jennifer needed the following adjustments for different activities:

- −30% for vacuuming

- −10% for grocery shopping

- −20% for raking leaves or scrubbing floors

On the flip side, an increase in basal rates may be needed for days with less activity. For example, Jennifer needed:

- +20% for riding in a car

- +30–50% for sick days

- It's best to get your temporary basal rate started at least 20 minutes before you start exercising. This will give your insulin level time to drop before you start.

- Some people choose to actually disconnect the pump from their body when they exercise. If you choose to follow this route, remember that when insulin levels get too low, you run the risk of ketoacidosis. So if your exercise session is going to be a long one, it's critical that you check for ketones.

■ For contact sports and prolonged activities, wearing a pump may not be very convenient. If this is the case, you might want to take an injection of glargine insulin to provide some basal insulin while you're not wearing the pump. See Chapter 12 for more on this.

The Practical Stuff

Infusion site care and selection for exercise

When you're going to be physically active with your pump, there are some things you need to keep in mind when it comes to your infusion set. The first is site location. Depending on the activity you have planned, you want to make sure your infusion set is in an area that won't get flexed or irritated. Too much bending or twisting may kink the cannula under your skin, or even pull it out of the site. So, if you're going to be swinging a baseball bat or golf club, you'll probably want to choose a site closer to the middle of your stomach, as opposed to somewhere on the "love handles." Somewhere on your hip might not be a bad option either.

You also want to be careful with the tubing. For example, if you're riding a bike and have your infusion set inserted in your thigh, you need to make sure the tubing has enough slack so that it doesn't pull out when you straighten your leg. Then again, you don't want so much slack that the tubing can get snagged on things and yanked out!

Make sure that the pump itself is away from the infusion site. This will prevent the pump from rubbing up against the infusion site. For example, if you have the infusion set inserted on the left side of your abdomen, simply clip the pump on the right side of your waistband.

Next you want to make sure the infusion set stays adhered to the site. Sweating from activity can loosen the attachment of the catheter to your skin. See the previous chapter for tips on how you can prevent this from happening.

Some Final Thoughts

As you begin exercising with the pump, keep in mind that every person responds differently to activity. Some people react differently to different activities. To figure out what works best for you, check your blood sugar frequently as you exercise. The guidelines we've talk about here are just a starting point. Your blood glucose records will give you the information you need for fine-tuning.

Meeting with an exercise physiologist who is trained in insulin pump therapy is your best bet for getting tight glucose control while exercising. Not only will an exercise physiologist be able to help you with advice on exercising safely, but he or she can also offer expert advice on unforeseen complications and how to achieve the best results from your activity.

In Chapter 12, we'll delve deeper into exercise and how it affects glucose metabolism and your own personal glucose control. As you move forward with your therapy, a more intense understanding of how exercise affects your body will help you tighten your control with the pump.

9 Keeping Track and Tracking Trouble

One of the most important aspects of successful pump therapy is knowing how to deal with unexpected problems. Without a doubt, you're going to run into situations that you didn't expect, and knowing how to handle them properly is very important. Of course troubleshooting skills don't appear after just a couple of days. More than likely, it will take a lot of practice and a lot of work with your diabetes care team. And there's no guarantee that you'll always be ready for what the pump throws your way. But, it's important that you have a good understanding of some of the more common problems and the guidelines you need to follow to keep these problems under control.

One thing most new pump users don't realize, however, is that the key to good troubleshooting is keeping good records. Yes, record keeping can be a nuisance and can be time consuming, but accurate and thorough record keeping is the key to successful pump therapy. How can you assess a problem if you don't know what factors have played a part? How can you notice a pattern if you haven't tracked your daily ups and downs? Knowing why something happened is the key to ensuring it doesn't happen again, and having detailed records is often the key to finding the answer.

So, before we get into what problems you might encounter and ways to handle them, let's talk about record keeping. This way, you can get a better idea of what you need to track and why you need to track it.

Record Keeping

We really can't stress the importance of good record keeping enough. It's virtually impossible to evaluate your progress and make meaningful adjustments to your insulin doses without accurate records of your blood glucose levels, food intake, and activity. Without this information, not only are you in the dark with what's happening, but so are your physicians and pump educators.

Many meters and pumps now offer downloadable records of your pump and meter activity. This is a great help in keeping accurate records, but it is no substitute for your own handwritten records, which are often referred to as *pump flowsheets*. More than likely, your physician or pump educator will provide you with pump flowsheets they prefer to work with. Your pump company will probably have flowsheets available as well. We've included some sample flowsheets in Appendix B. They might not be exactly like the ones you'll use, but they should give you a pretty good idea of what information needs to be recorded and how it needs to be organized.

So, what kinds of information should you record in your pump flowsheet?

What to record?

When it comes to record keeping, the more detailed the better. Very rarely is someone on the pump accused of recording too much in his or her pump records. Of course, you don't want to overwhelm yourself with so much information that the accuracy of your records starts to slip. A ton of information can be useless (or even confusing) if it's not recorded accurately. For example, let's say you're looking at your records and you notice that there's a significant drop in your blood glucose from one reading to the next. You might think that it's time to lower your basal rate. However, the real problem is that you forgot to record a bolus dose between your readings.

So the message is simple. Record everything that matters, and record it as accurately as you can. The following list details some of the things you'll want to include in your pump flowsheets:

- Blood glucose measurements
- Basal rate(s)
- Carbohydrate intake
- Specific foods eaten (be sure to record *all* foods eaten, especially at first)
- Where foods are eaten—home vs. restaurant
- Food boluses
- Correction boluses
- Activity or exercise—type, length, and intensity
- Work hours—especially if you work varied shifts
- Day of the week
- When you change your infusion set
- How you feel—sick, highly stressed, etc.
- Any symptoms of hypoglycemia (especially if you have hypoglycemia unawareness)
- Time of month, in relation to your menstrual cycle
- Medications

Of course, there may be additional things that you or your physician would like to note in your records. Talk with your diabetes care team about what needs to be included on your pump flowsheet.

When to record?

The best way to keep your records accurate is to record things when they happen. Saying you'll write it down later or waiting for a "more convenient time" just gives you time to forget details and opens the door to mistakes. If you want to keep your records accurate, it's best that you *keep your pump flowsheet with you at all times.* Some people like to set aside a few minutes every day for recording things, which is okay if you're willing to use the stored information in your meter and pump. However, try not to go longer than 1 day without keeping written records. Your pump and meter may have infallible memories, but you may not be able to say the same thing about yourself!

Most of your detailed record keeping will take place in the first several months of pump therapy. After awhile, when you're comfortable with your basal rates and bolus doses, you'll be able to take occasional breaks from record keeping. You probably won't need to be as detailed either. However, there's a chance that you'll want to shift your focus to more specific areas of your therapy, such as exercise, and keep detailed records in that area. Keep in mind that you'll never want to abandon record keeping completely. If from time to time your therapy is not as tight as you'd like, detailed record keeping is the first step to getting back on track.

Pump Flowsheets

In Appendix B at the end of this book, you'll find some sample pump flowsheets you can study to get a better idea of what a flowsheet will look like and what you'll want to record. Your physician may even suggest copying these flowsheets for your own records. Or, he or she may provide some flowsheets that he or she prefers. More than likely, however, these flowsheets will vary in appearance rather than information.

The first flowsheet is meant to be kept per day and is designed to help you focus on what food you've eaten and the carb content of each item. Because it allows room for detailed food records, this one is particularly helpful if you plan to meet with a Registered Dietitian and are looking for ways to control your weight.

The second flowsheet is designed to record 2 days worth of information. While there's not a specific place dedicated to foods, there's plenty of room to list the foods you ate in the space below each day's record.

The third flowsheet is designed for the more advanced pump users who would like to fit 4 days worth of records onto 1 sheet. These sheets also make it easier to analyze trends over long periods of time—less sheets to look at!

Which sheet is right for you depends on where you are in your pump therapy and what information is important to you. Keep in mind that these aren't the only pump flowsheets available and that your situation may even call for a custom flowsheet to better meet your needs. You and your diabetes care team will be able to determine what flowsheet will work best for you.

When Chaos Strikes—The Art of Troubleshooting

It's easy to assume that once you have your basal rates, bolus doses, and carbohydrate counting down, you have the pump pretty much figured out. Unfortunately, it's not quite that simple. While these aspects make up most of pump therapy, you always have to be ready for the unexpected. Keeping good records is a way to help cope with these unforeseen events; you can check your records, look for patterns or inconsistencies, and work out a solution. There are always going to be swings and fluctuations that keep you out of your target range, and having a good idea what can cause these swings can keep you on the right track.

In the rest of this chapter, we'll talk about some of the common unexpected problems, what causes them, and how you can handle them. We'll talk about what to do when you have high blood sugars, low blood sugars, and sick days. More than likely, you'll encounter situations that aren't covered in this chapter, and at these times, the expertise of your physician and pump educators, as well as experience that you have gained, will be your best tools for coming up with a solution.

Troubleshooting Hyperglycemia

Before you started pump therapy, or considered starting pump therapy, you learned about some of the more common causes of high blood sugar, such as illness and stress. While these causes still hold true for pump therapy, you'll find that the pump also brings its own unique causes of hyperglycemia, including:

- A kinked or dislodged catheter (the number 1 cause)
- Infection at your infusion site
- Your pump running out of insulin
- Pump failure
- Your batteries running down
- A clogged catheter
- Air bubbles in your tubing

As with all insulin therapy, your goal in pump therapy is to avoid hyperglycemia; high blood sugar is easier to prevent than it is to treat. However, if you are on the pump and hyperglycemia does strike, you must treat it seriously and with immediate action. Because your pump uses only fast-acting insulin, you're much more susceptible to diabetic ketoacidosis than someone using a combination of fast- and long-acting insulins. Any interruption of your insulin delivery from the pump can lead to high blood sugars very quickly.

Causes of Hyperglycemia

Common causes
- Illness
- Stress
- Insulin deficiency
- Too much food

Pump-related causes
- Kinked or dislodged catheter
- Infection at infusion site
- Pump out of insulin
- Pump failure
- New batteries needed
- Clogged catheter
- Air bubbles in tubing

> ### Action Steps to Treat "Common/Explained" Hyperglycemia
>
> 1. If your high blood sugars can be attributed to a common cause, such as forgetting to bolus at a meal or eating too much food, simply use your Sensitivity Factor to determine a correction dose and then bolus.
> 2. Recheck your blood glucose in 2 hours if you're using Humalog/Novolog, or 4 hours if you're using regular/Velosulin to make sure your glucose levels are dropping.

What to do when you have "unexplained" hyperglycemia

If you find yourself with hyperglycemia that *cannot* be related to a common cause—illness, miscalculated carb content, overeating, etc.—then you should consider it *unexplained hyperglycemia*. Follow the steps below:

- If your blood glucose level is 250 mg/dl or higher, check your urine or blood for ketones immediately!
- Refer to Figure 9-1, "Guidelines for Supplemental Insulin," for guidance on how much insulin to take and how you should take it.
- Refer to Figure 9-2, "Troubleshooting the Pump," to see what steps you need to take to identify a possible cause for your unexplained high blood sugars.
- Drink plenty of sugar-free fluids to avoid dehydration from your high blood glucose.
- *Contact your health care provider* if there is no improvement in high blood glucose after *2 supplemental insulin doses.*

> ### Remember!
>
> If you have "unexplained" hyperglycemia, immediately follow these 4 steps in order:
>
> **Step 1:** Check ketone levels to determine the amount of insulin you will need.
> **Step 2:** Take insulin to correct the hyperglycemia.
> **Step 3:** Troubleshoot the cause of the problem (see Fig. 9-2).
> **Step 4:** If you still can't find the source of the problem, change your infusion set.

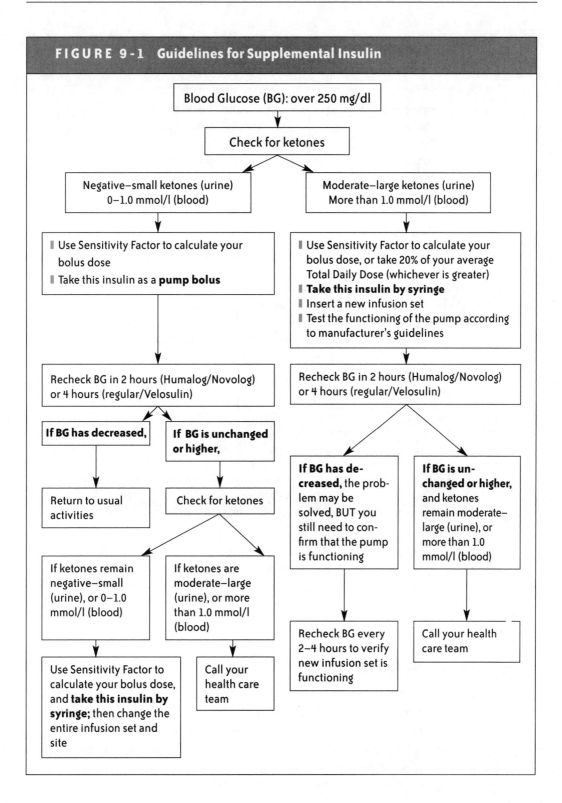

FIGURE 9-1   Guidelines for Supplemental Insulin

Blood Glucose (BG): over 250 mg/dl

Check for ketones

Negative–small ketones (urine)
0–1.0 mmol/l (blood)

- Use Sensitivity Factor to calculate your bolus dose
- Take this insulin as a **pump bolus**

Recheck BG in 2 hours (Humalog/Novolog) or 4 hours (regular/Velosulin)

If BG has decreased,

If BG is unchanged or higher,

Return to usual activities

Check for ketones

If ketones remain negative–small (urine), or 0–1.0 mmol/l (blood)

If ketones are moderate–large (urine), or more than 1.0 mmol/l (blood)

Use Sensitivity Factor to calculate your bolus dose, and **take this insulin by syringe;** then change the entire infusion set and site

Call your health care team

Moderate–large ketones (urine)
More than 1.0 mmol/l (blood)

- Use Sensitivity Factor to calculate your bolus dose, or take 20% of your average Total Daily Dose (whichever is greater)
- **Take this insulin by syringe**
- Insert a new infusion set
- Test the functioning of the pump according to manufacturer's guidelines

Recheck BG in 2 hours (Humalog/Novolog) or 4 hours (regular/Velosulin)

If BG has decreased, the problem may be solved, BUT you still need to confirm that the pump is functioning

If BG is unchanged or higher, and ketones remain moderate–large (urine), or more than 1.0 mmol/l (blood)

Recheck BG every 2–4 hours to verify new infusion set is functioning

Call your health care team

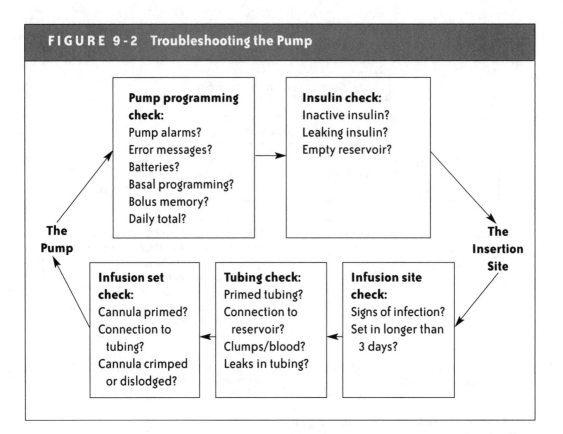

FIGURE 9-2   Troubleshooting the Pump

Pump programming check:
Pump alarms?
Error messages?
Batteries?
Basal programming?
Bolus memory?
Daily total?

Insulin check:
Inactive insulin?
Leaking insulin?
Empty reservoir?

The Pump

The Insertion Site

Infusion set check:
Cannula primed?
Connection to tubing?
Cannula crimped or dislodged?

Tubing check:
Primed tubing?
Connection to reservoir?
Clumps/blood?
Leaks in tubing?

Infusion site check:
Signs of infection?
Set in longer than 3 days?

Smart Pumping Tip

When in doubt, change it out!
If you have unexplained blood glucose readings of 250 mg/dl or more 2 times in a row, change the cartridge and infusion set and check for ketones. Take fast-acting insulin as directed by your health care professional.

Some facts about ketones

DKA can develop much more rapidly if you're on the pump and can be life-threatening. The good news is that, although this condition is serious, it is preventable. As a pump user, you need to be constantly aware that unexplained high blood sugar arising from insufficient insulin that is not immediately treated can rapidly turn into DKA.

Caution!

There are no long-acting insulins used in pump therapy, so any accidental interruption of insulin delivery can quickly lead to diabetic ketoacidosis!

Having a better understanding of how this process plays itself out in your body will help you avoid the possibility of DKA.

- Insulin plays a key role in controlling the production of glucose and ketones by your liver.
- When insulin levels in the bloodstream drop, this triggers your liver to start producing ketones and glucose. Your liver mistakenly "thinks" that the low insulin levels mean you need more energy. As a result, the glucose and ketone levels in your bloodstream rise.

Caution!

Nausea is an early sign of DKA. If you're feeling nauseated or sick to your stomach, check for ketones.

To Prevent DKA

- Check your blood glucose at least 4 times a day—DKA can develop much faster if you're on the pump.

- If you have "unexplained" hyperglycemia (250 mg/dl or higher), immediately check for ketones.

- Take supplemental insulin to lower your high blood glucose levels.

- Drink plenty of fluids to avoid dehydration.

Always carry:

- Insulin and a syringe, or an insulin pen

- A blood glucose meter and strips

- Ketone strips

- An extra infusion set and reservoir

- Extra batteries for your pump and meter

■ Ketones are acidic, and as they build up in your bloodstream, your blood becomes more acidic. This is known as *acidosis*.

■ The kidneys start to "filter" the glucose and ketones from the blood, which causes increased urination. This extra loss of fluids can lead to dehydration.

■ The increased urination can also lead to a loss of *electrolytes*, such as sodium, potassium, and phosphate. This can lead to a chemical imbalance in the body.

Troubleshooting Hypoglycemia

As a person with diabetes, you've undoubtedly had episodes of hypoglycemia. Inevitably, any person with diabetes looking for tight glucose control is going to occasionally dip down below their target range into a hypoglycemic reaction.

What many find surprising is that the human body is designed to avoid hypoglycemic reactions, with a variety of safeguards built in to keep your blood sugar from dropping dangerously low. Unfortunately, this system is disrupted within a few years of being diagnosed with type 1 diabetes. Ultimately, your body's only immediate response to a low blood sugar reaction is a rush of *epinephrine*, or adrenaline. This epinephrine triggers the liver to release glucose into the blood and also causes shakiness and rapid heartbeat, which are signals to you to eat some food and get your glucose levels back up to normal. Unfortunately, people who suffer frequent hypoglycemia can even lose this safeguard (hypoglycemia unawareness).

If you've ever used insulin before, you've been made well aware of the dangers of low blood sugars. You know *why* you should avoid hypoglycemia. The tricky part is *how* you avoid hypoglycemia.

Halting hypoglycemia

The best defense against hypoglycemia is to try to identify the situations that can result in low blood sugar, understand why they happen, and know what you can do to avoid or treat the problem.

Frequently checking your blood sugar is the best method of keeping hypoglycemia at bay. This allows you to catch a dip in blood glucose levels before it even produces symptoms. If you have hypoglycemia unawareness, this may be your only method of managing low blood sugar without serious repercussions.

Different people respond to low blood sugar differently and at different levels. Some may notice symptoms when their blood glucose is 65 mg/dl; others may not notice until their blood sugar is 50 mg/dl. But no matter what, *always* treat a low blood sugar *as soon* as you notice symptoms. Having a plan makes this treatment much more effective and helps guard against "over-treating," which usually results in *hyper*glycemia later on. The following is a step-by-step approach to treating hypoglycemia.

> **Smart Pumping Tip**
>
> **Rule of 15 for hypoglycemia:**
>
> ▍ Consume 15 grams of quick-acting carbohydrate.
>
> ▍ Wait 15 minutes; recheck your blood glucose.
>
> ▍ If glucose level is <80 mg/dl, repeat above.

Steps for treating hypoglycemia

Step 1: If possible, confirm your hypoglycemia by checking your blood glucose.

Step 2: Treat immediately with 15–20 grams of carbohydrate if:

- Your BG is less than 80 mg/dl and you are experiencing symptoms.

> **Good Sources of Carb**
>
> When looking for carb to treat hypoglycemia, it's best to use a form that will absorb quickly. Foods that can be directly absorbed in your mouth, such as glucose tablets, syrup, or honey, will work the quickest. Avoid foods that are high in fat, as they tend to slow your absorption of carbohydrate. The following foods and drinks will supply the 15 grams of carb you need to counteract a low blood glucose:
>
> ▍ 3–4 glucose tablets or gel (works fastest)
>
> ▍ 1 tablespoon of honey or maple syrup
>
> ▍ 5–6 Lifesaver candies
>
> ▍ 4–6 oz of regular soda
>
> ▍ 4 oz of fruit juice
>
> ▍ 2 tablespoons of raisins
>
> ▍ 8 oz of nonfat or 1% milk

■ Your BG is less than 70 mg/dl with or without symptoms.

Step 3: Recheck your BG in 15 minutes.

■ If your BG is less than 80 mg/dl, repeat Steps 2 and 3.
■ If your BG is more than 80 mg/dl, continue with Step 4.

Step 4: Consider the timing of your last bolus and your activity—then decide if you need further treatment.

Step 5: Try to figure out the cause of the hypoglycemia so you can prevent it in the future (see below).

Possible causes of hypoglycemia

There are a variety of factors that can lead to hypoglycemia. Following is a list of some of the more common causes:

■ Miscalculation of bolus
■ Overlapping bolus doses
■ Increased activity or exercise
■ Lag effect of exercise
■ Inaccurate programming of your pump
■ Basal rate set too high
■ Target blood glucose level set too low
■ Alcohol

Additional things to consider with hypoglycemia

■ *Do not* suspend your insulin pump delivery during an episode of hypoglycemia.
■ Train a member of your family or a significant other to use a *glucagon emergency kit*, and make sure that your kit has not expired. This will be necessary if you're suffering from severe hypoglycemia that can lead to unconsciousness.
■ If you have recurrent, unexplained hypoglycemia, contact your diabetes care team.
■ If you have changes in your usual activity or are drinking alcohol, check your blood glucose levels more frequently.

Managing "Sick Days"

As you've probably discovered, when you're sick your blood glucose can become more difficult to manage, and often results in high blood glucose levels. Thus, you often hear a lot about "sick days" as adverse situations that can affect your diabetes management. However, the term "sick day" has come to mean much more than just a day you're a little under the weather. Now it covers a broad range of conditions that can lead to rising blood glucose, such as:

- Major stress
- Infections
- Common cold
- Flu
- Injury
- Invasive dental work
- Severe emotional trauma

So what do all of these situations have in common? Basically, your body responds to the stress of any of the above by releasing *stress hormones*. These hormones trigger your liver to release glucose into your bloodstream, while at the same time causing your body's cells to become less sensitive (responsive) to insulin. What you get in the end is rising blood glucose even if you aren't eating. In addition, these stress hormones trigger your liver to release ketones, which, left unchecked, will

Stress and Your Diabetes: Some Pump Management Tips

Stress can have a powerful impact on your blood glucose levels. When you are feeling stressed, your body releases hormones that can swing your blood glucose wildly. These fluctuations can make your therapy seem like a frustrating battle that just leads to more stress. The impact stress has on glucose management can vary from person to person, which makes it hard to offer specific guidelines. There are, however, some pointers:

- A corrective bolus will usually manage the highs that follow momentary anxiety.

- Your basal rate may need to be increased for more prolonged periods of stress, such as when a family member is ill.

- A temporary basal rate increase will sometimes be effective for repeated stresses (such as work meetings!) that usually raise your glucose levels.

lead to DKA. This is why it's so important to check your blood glucose and ketones frequently on sick days. Having an *action plan* can also help immensely.

Action plan for sick days

1. Contact your health care provider for guidance.
2. *Always* take your insulin—your blood glucose can rise quickly.
3. Even if you can't eat, *do not* stop taking your basal dose. You may even find that you need more insulin than usual.
4. Check your blood glucose every 2–3 hours, day and night, and record your results.
5. Check your urine (or blood) for ketones if your blood glucose is 250 mg/dl or higher.
6. Take extra insulin if your blood glucose is 250 mg/dl or higher. See Figure 9-1, "Guidelines for Supplemental Insulin," on page 99 for guidance on how much insulin to take and how to take it.
7. Drink plenty of decaffeinated fluids, day and night, to prevent dehydration:

   - Drink 8 oz of fluid every 30–60 minutes
   - If you are able to eat, drink water or diet soda
   - If you can't eat, alternate calorie-containing fluids with non-calorie fluids every 30–60 minutes

8. Feed your body. Try to eat some foods with carbohydrate in small amounts throughout the day for extra energy. Good choices include:

   - 1/2 cup applesauce, pudding, cooked cereal, or regular Jell-O
   - 4–6 oz of regular soda, such as ginger ale or cola
   - 6 saltines or a slice of toast

Moving Forward

So we've covered the basics. By now you should have a pretty good understanding of how the pump works, how to adjust your insulin dose, and how to handle pump therapy during adverse situations. We've seen some of the common problems and offered ways to resolve them. For all intents and purposes, we've covered the majority of information you need to know about day-to-day insulin pump therapy.

However, as diabetes has probably shown you, most days are not average days, and knowing the basics will only get you so far. If you really want tight control (which you probably do—you made the move to the pump didn't you?), you're going to need more than just basics.

In the next section, we'll cover some of the more advanced concepts that are associated with intensive therapy. We'll talk about how insulin works and what factors will affect how well your insulin works. We'll discuss nutrition in depth, as well as more about exercising safely and effectively with the pump.

III

Beyond the Basics:
Intensive Management
and Pump Use
In the Real World

10 Understanding Insulin:
How It Acts and How You Respond

As you've probably noticed, understanding insulin and how your body responds to insulin can be a tricky endeavor. Often times, you may feel there's a wide gap between how an insulin is supposed to act and how that insulin really acts in your body. Sometimes, the action profiles are right on; other times, your reaction can seem sluggish and painfully slow. This can make getting tight control seem like an impossible feat.

In this chapter, we'll talk about how the insulin you take is supposed to act by detailing some insulin profiles and give you some pointers for refining your insulin boluses and basal rates. We'll also discuss some of the outside factors that can affect your bolus doses and basal rates and try to take some of the mystery out of the fluctuating responses to insulin you may have. You may find that some of the issues we discuss relate directly to you, while some may not apply to your situation at all. Every pump user is different, and what works for others may not work for you.

Remember, having a good understanding of insulin and your own sensitivity (responsiveness) to insulin is a major component of good, tight diabetes management. Unfortunately, a book can only give you so much information and cannot be tailored to your individual situation. We can, however, present information that can push you to explore options and discuss issues of which you may not have been aware. Using the following information and working closely with your diabetes care team can bring you a lot closer to your diabetes management goals.

Getting the Most Out of Your Insulin

Remember the action profile of insulin

In a fully functioning endocrine system, the pancreas releases insulin directly into the bloodstream, which means the insulin can get to where it needs to go and make an impact rather quickly. For people with diabetes, insulin must be injected and then absorbed from the fat underneath the skin before it can take effect. This means that the insulin you receive from your pump will take much longer to get to work and have an impact on your blood glucose levels.

Figure 10-1 is an illustration of an *action profile* for both regular insulin and Humalog insulin. No doubt you've seen action profiles for insulin before. These figures represent how long it takes your body to

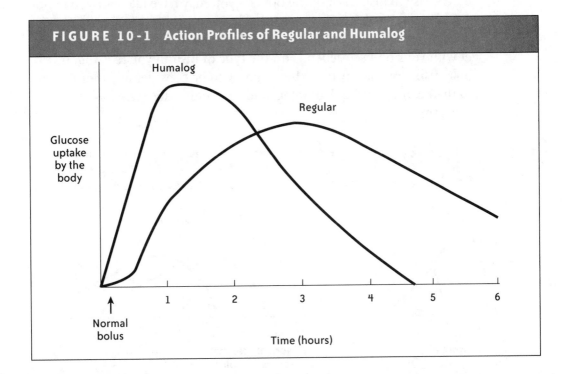

FIGURE 10-1   Action Profiles of Regular and Humalog

absorb insulin and how long this insulin remains active in your bloodstream after a bolus or injection. As you can see, Humalog insulin is absorbed much faster than regular insulin. This is because Humalog has a slight chemical modification that allows it to be absorbed more quickly.

Beware of overlapping boluses!

Once you move forward with your pump therapy, you'll soon find that knowing the action profile of your insulin is extremely important. In fact, it's almost impossible to effectively calculate and administer a bolus dose without considering the action profile of your insulin. For example, let's say you check your blood glucose level and find that you're running a little high. There are no ketones present, so you're not in a crisis situation. You use your Sensitivity Factor (SF) to determine a correction bolus and bolus your insulin to get your glucose levels down. Two hours later, you check your blood glucose again and find that you're still running a little bit high. Understandably, you want to bolus again. However, since you just bolused 2 hours ago, you need to be familiar with the action profile of your insulin to see what kind of overlap you're going to get. It's easy to lose track of the boluses you may have taken; if you're not sure, check the bolus history recorded by your pump.

As you can see from Figure 10-2, how much overlap you're going to get with your boluses depends on the type of insulin you're using. If you're using regular insulin, there's going to be considerably more overlap than if you're using Humalog, and your bolus dose will have to reflect this.

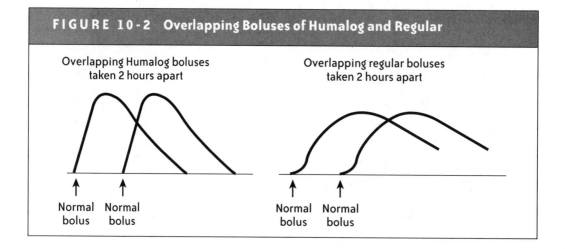

FIGURE 10-2   Overlapping Boluses of Humalog and Regular

Overlapping Humalog boluses
taken 2 hours apart

Overlapping regular boluses
taken 2 hours apart

Normal   Normal
bolus   bolus

Normal   Normal
bolus   bolus

You also need to keep in mind that the *larger your bolus is, the longer the action profile of your insulin will be*. Larger doses of insulin are absorbed more slowly by your body and will remain active much longer than smaller doses, especially with regular insulin. As illustrated in Figure 10-3, you can see that with regular insulin, there's a marked increase in action profile duration as the size of the bolus increases. Note that this lengthening of the action profile is not as dramatic with Humalog.

Understanding the lengthened action profiles of bigger boluses is especially necessary if you are less sensitive (responsive) to insulin and require larger doses to control your diabetes. If you also use regular insulin, as opposed to Humalog/Novolog, your likelihood of overlapping boluses increases even more. If you use regular insulin, and in larger amounts than most, you must be very careful with your second bolus dose. So, before you take any bolus dose, *always remember the action profile of your insulin*. If your previous bolus is still active and your blood glucose is still high, you'll need to play it safe and take less than your calculated dose. High blood sugar is a problem, but try not to let your desire to keep your blood sugars under control send you into a hypoglycemic reaction.

Which insulin should I use in my pump?

Up until the fall of 2001, when Novolog was introduced, choices were pretty limited for pump users. Since pumps only use fast-acting insulin, choices consisted of Humalog or regular (a special formulation, Velosulin Buffered Regular, was also available for use in pumps). Of the 2, Humalog has proven to be the most popular choice for insulin pump users for a variety of reasons. The advantages of Humalog include:

- An action profile that more closely mimics the insulin secreted by your pancreas.
- More rapid absorption, which means there's no need to bolus ahead of meals, and high blood glucose can be brought down much more quickly.
- Shorter action profile, which means there's less chance of hypoglycemia several hours after a meal.

You'll notice that the last advantage of Humalog is a shorter action profile that lessens the risk of hypoglycemia several hours after a meal. For people who tend to suffer from low blood glucose levels in the early hours of the morning, this is a big bonus. Because regular insulin tends to remain active much longer than Humalog, the "tail" of the supper bolus will still be active well into the evening, driving blood sugars down in the early hours of the morning. If you eat supper close to bedtime and tend to use large doses of insulin, this effect can be even more dramatic (we'll talk more about nighttime blood sugar management later in this chapter).

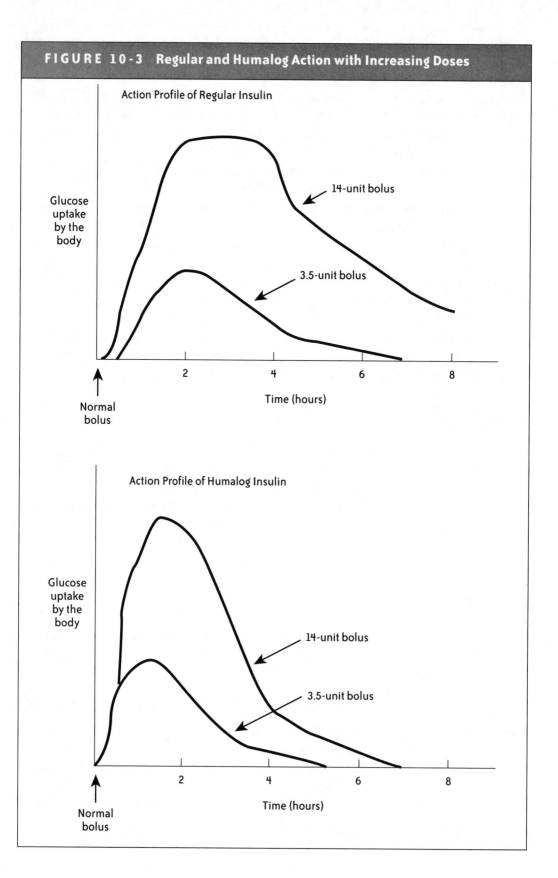

FIGURE 10-3   Regular and Humalog Action with Increasing Doses

Action Profile of Regular Insulin

Glucose uptake by the body

14-unit bolus

3.5-unit bolus

2   4   6   8

Time (hours)

Normal bolus

Action Profile of Humalog Insulin

Glucose uptake by the body

14-unit bolus

3.5-unit bolus

2   4   6   8

Time (hours)

Normal bolus

Of course, Humalog also has some downsides. Some disadvantages of Humalog include:

- More rapid absorption. Yeah, we know, just a second ago we said it was an advantage, and it is. However, this rapid absorption also has some negative aspects, such as:

  - A greater risk for rapidly appearing hyperglycemia and diabetic ketoacidosis if there is any interruption of insulin from the pump.
  - The possibility that insulin can start acting before the glucose in your meal is absorbed, which can lead to hypoglycemia 1–2 hours after you eat your meal. This is generally limited to times when your pre-meal BG is below 100 mg/dl and you eat a meal in which the carbs are absorbed very slowly, such as a meal high in fat. Taking your bolus after your meal or using the "square wave/extended" bolus feature (which is available on some pumps) usually solves this problem.

- Poor stability in pumps. Right now, Humalog is *not* approved by the Food and Drug Administration for use in pumps. Although clinical studies have indicated that Humalog is fine for insulin pumps, some people have reported problems with Humalog that were resolved by changing to another type of insulin. In rare cases, Humalog has precipitated in pump infusion catheters. If you would like to see a photograph of a catheter in which Humalog has precipitated, as well as case studies where this occurred, you can visit the website for the *British Medical Journal* at *http://www.bmj.com/cgi/reprint/324/7348/1253.pdf.* Your health care provider can also provide you with more information.

There's no data documenting how often pump users experience problems with Humalog instability, so it's not really known how common the problem really is. Our experience has shown that such instability is quite rare. However, there is a small group of people on the pump using Humalog who have noticed that their blood glucose tends to rise 1–2 days after changing their infusion sets. This problem is usually resolved by changing infusion sets more often or by switching to Novolog or Velosulin Buffered Regular insulin.

Novolog, which was introduced in the fall of 2001, *has* been approved by the Food and Drug Administration for use in insulin pumps. Published data suggests that Novolog and Humalog have similar action profiles, though some have noted a difference when changing from one to the other.

Do Humalog, Novolog, and regular insulin have the same potency?

Contrary to what many people think, all 3 insulins have about the same potency. One unit of Humalog will stimulate the tissues of your body to take up as much glucose as 1 unit of regular or 1 unit of Novolog. This means that in principle, your Insulin-to-Carbohydrate ratio and SF should remain the same if you switch from one insulin to another (there are unexplained cases of patients experiencing different potency levels between insulins, but these cases are rare). However, because Humalog and Novolog pack their punch into a much shorter period, over-bolusing these insulins will send your glucose plummeting much more rapidly than regular insulin.

Are there any factors that can affect insulin absorption from the catheter site?

Yes, there are a few things that can affect how well your insulin is absorbed and how quickly it can start lowering your blood glucose. These include:

- Where the catheter is placed on your body. Insulin is generally absorbed faster in the abdomen. However, if you're exercising, blood flow to your legs will increase and insulin will be absorbed much quicker here than usual. If you're a runner, you may want to avoid placing the infusion catheter in your thigh.
- The amount of *subcutaneous fat*. Subcutaneous fat is just another way to describe the fat underneath your skin. If you place your catheter in a place where there's more subcutaneous fat, insulin will be absorbed slower. Some pump users have noticed the area in the middle of their abdomen absorbs at a different rate than the side of their abdomen.
- How much scarring there is at the infusion site. Using the same site over and over leads to scarring, and this will cause the insulin to be absorbed slower. Inserting the catheter near a surgical scar will also lead to irregular absorption.
- Temperature. Heat can make your blood vessels dilate, or become larger, which increases the flow of blood. This can cause insulin to be absorbed more quickly. If you find yourself going low after some time in a whirlpool, sauna, or hot shower, this may be why.

> **Caution!**
>
> If you're already a pump user and you'll be switching to another brand of pump, the dosage may differ, so it's probably wise to check your blood glucose more often.

■ Traveling in high altitudes. Some pump users have experienced problems while traveling in areas of high altitude, such as the mountains. If you'll be traveling in such an area, it would probably be best to do extra blood glucose checks to make sure things are okay.

Factors that Affect Your Basal and Bolus Requirements

As you move forward with your pump therapy, you'll notice that the same basal rates and bolus doses won't work all the time every day. Your insulin needs tend to be different at different times of the day and from one day to the next. Because of this, taking advantage of different basal rates and making adjustments to your bolus doses can be a big help in keeping your blood glucose levels in check. Of course, these varying insulin requirements differ from person to person. However, there is one time of the day that affects almost every adolescent and adult with diabetes in the same way—nighttime.

Controlling your glucose overnight

When it comes to controlling your blood glucose overnight, we must once again turn to controlling the actions of the liver. As we've mentioned, the liver acts as a glucose reservoir, releasing glucose into your bloodstream between meals and while you sleep. During these periods, insulin must be present in your bloodstream or else your liver will produce too much glucose and ketones, and you'll end up with hyperglycemia and maybe even ketoacidosis. This is why you use basal insulin—to regulate blood glucose during those times when you're not eating. If you don't have enough basal insulin while you sleep, you wake up in the morning with high blood sugar.

While there are a lucky few who can use the same basal pattern all day and all night, most people on the pump will need several different basal rates to effectively control their glucose levels overnight. The most typical pattern for adolescents and adults (but not children) is as follows:

1. Late at night and in the early hours of the morning (11 P.M.–2 A.M.), your body will often be *more* sensitive (responsive) to insulin. During this time, you will need a lower basal rate than usual. If you plan to correct for high blood glucose during this period, you will also need to use a smaller bolus dose than your usual SF indicates. A correction bolus based on your usual SF could send you into hypoglycemia.

> **Caution!**
>
> If you take a correction bolus at bedtime, you may need to bolus less than your usual Sensitivity Factor indicates. Because of increased sensitivity to insulin, your usual correction bolus could lead to hypoglycemia.

2. As the night goes on, your insulin needs will probably move in the opposite direction. During the period right before dawn, from about 3–5 A.M. until 8–9 A.M., your body will often be *less* sensitive to insulin. This is known as the *dawn phenomenon*, a condition related to the production of growth hormone by your body. Since your body will be *less* sensitive to insulin, you'll need to set your basal rate a little bit *higher* than normal during this period to keep your glucose levels down. The dawn phenomenon occurs at different times for each person, so the period in which you'll need to up your basal rate will be different from others. This will be something you need to work out with your diabetes care team. In addition, the dawn phenomenon will be more severe from person to person and can fluctuate in severity from day to day. Some people won't even experience the dawn phenomenon at all and, thus, will not need to change their basal rate. Keep in mind that if you *do* experience a change in your sensitivity during the early hours of the morning, you may need to take more insulin than normal to cover your breakfast carbohydrates.

Other factors that affect your basal rates and bolus doses

While nighttime fluctuations can often be the most dramatic, as well as the most common, there are other factors that can cause your glucose levels to swing in unexpected ways. The following factors are things you need to keep in mind when you're analyzing your blood glucose:

- The delayed effects of exercise and physical activity
- The "rebound" effect from hypoglycemia
- The impact of hyperglycemia on your insulin sensitivity
- The impact of high-fat foods and caffeine on your insulin sensitivity
- The impact of certain medications
- The impact of your menstrual cycle, if you're a woman
- The impact of certain medical conditions

Alcohol can also have quite an impact on your body's sensitivity to insulin. We'll talk more about this in the next chapter when we talk about nutrition. Also remember that if your weight or level of physical activity changes, your insulin sensitivity will change as well (Fig. 10-4).

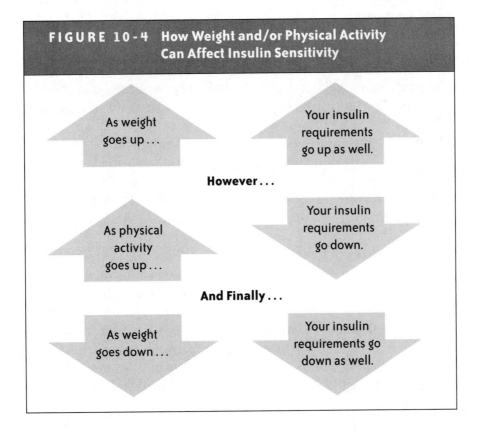

FIGURE 10-4   How Weight and/or Physical Activity Can Affect Insulin Sensitivity

As weight goes up...

Your insulin requirements go up as well.

However...

As physical activity goes up...

Your insulin requirements go down.

And Finally...

As weight goes down...

Your insulin requirements go down as well.

The delayed effects of physical activity

We'll talk more about the effects of weight and exercise on your insulin requirements in Chapter 12. For now, keep in mind that exercise or prolonged physical activity can continue to affect your blood glucose levels well after you've finished being active. During physical activity, the glucose that's stored in your muscles is used up. To replenish this lost glucose, your muscles will pull glucose from the blood, dropping your overall blood glucose levels. Depending on how active you were, this impact can last for anywhere between a few hours to a day and a half. If you were active in the evening, you may need to lower your usual nighttime basal rate to avoid hypoglycemia.

"Rebound" from hypoglycemia

Often times after a hypoglycemic episode, your blood glucose levels will rise higher than expected. This is known as a hypoglycemic *rebound*. There are a couple of ways this rebound can happen. One is through your body's own defense mechanisms. The other is through over-treatment on your part.

- **Natural rebound.** Your body has a number of hormonal defenses against hypoglycemia. When you have a hypoglycemic reaction, several hormones (including epinephrine, growth hormone, and cortisol) are produced and released into your bloodstream. These hormones trigger your liver to produce glucose, while at the same time lowering your sensitivity to insulin. The result is high blood sugar. This rebound increase in blood sugar usually lasts a few hours, but sometimes may last for over a day.
- **Over-treatment rebound.** Because it usually takes a little while for your body to absorb the carb you eat when you have a low blood sugar, there's a tendency to over-treat the condition. It's natural to want to keep eating carb until your glucose levels are normal and overcompensation is common. Unfortunately, this can catch up with you in the end, resulting in high blood sugars. How much carb you should eat to counteract your low blood glucose depends on your situation and how low your blood glucose is. It's best to use forms of carb that you can absorb directly through your mouth, such as maple syrup or glucose tablets. These will act more quickly, so there's less of a tendency to overeat.

Caution!

A "rebound" from a hypoglycemic episode while you're sleeping can make your morning glucose levels even higher than normal. Indications of a nighttime hypoglycemic episode include nightmares, restless sleep, sweat and/or damp nightclothes, and a headache in the morning.

Hyperglycemia and your insulin sensitivity

When blood glucose levels get very high, your sensitivity to insulin will probably drop. This means that the Sensitivity Factor you use to drop ordinary high blood glucose probably won't be accurate for very high blood glucose.

   For example, if you have an SF of 40, then it's expected that 1 unit of insulin will drop your blood glucose by 40 mg/dl—from 160 mg/dl to 120 mg/dl. However, if your glucose is very high, let's say around 280 mg/dl, then your body will be less sensitive to insulin and that 1 unit

---

Insulin Adjustments for Very High Blood Glucose

Rikki and her diabetes care team analyze her blood glucose records. They find if her Blood Glucose (BG) is 220 mg/dl or less, her SF of 40 works just fine. However, when her glucose rises above 220 mg/dl, her correction dose doesn't bring her down to her target BG of 100 mg/dl.

Her physician gives her the following guidelines:

▌ Calculate correction dose using regular SF.

▌ If BG is 220–260 mg/dl, take calculated dose *plus* 0.5 units.

▌ If BG is 261–300 mg/dl, take calculated dose *plus* 1 unit.

▌ If BG is 301–340 mg/dl, take calculated dose *plus* 2 units.

Using these guidelines, Rikki calculates her correction dose for 2 different BG levels.

1. At 200 mg/dl, she determines she would take 2.5 units of insulin (200 – 100 = 100/40 = 2.5), since she doesn't need to add any extra insulin.

2. At 280 mg/dl, she determines she would take 5.5 units of insulin (280 – 100 = 180/40 = 4.5 + 1), since she needs to add 1 unit to her correction when her BG is this high.

of insulin won't lower your glucose as much. Instead of lowering your BG 40 mg/dl, it may just lower it 20–30 mg/dl.

Scan your glucose records. Do you find that your Sensitivity Factor works well when the glucose level is in the 100's but doesn't work as well when you're in the 200's? If this sounds familiar, you may need to add extra insulin to your correction bolus when you're running very high. Talk with your diabetes care team about this change in sensitivity as your glucose levels get higher. They should be able to develop a Sensitivity Factor that can help you with your insulin adjustment.

However, you probably will *not* need to take extra insulin if you're correcting at bedtime. Remember that at this time, you're probably more sensitive to insulin and may need to take even less than normal.

Foods and your insulin sensitivity

We'll talk more about nutrition and what foods can affect your blood glucose in the next chapter. For now, keep the following in mind:

- High-fat foods can reduce your sensitivity to insulin. Any meal with a lot of fat may call for an insulin adjustment in your food bolus.
- Caffeine can reduce your sensitivity as well. If you have a cup of coffee with your meal, you'll probably need to up your food bolus a little.

The impact of medications

Different medications have different impacts on your glucose levels. Before you take any medication, consult with your diabetes care team to see how this new medicine can affect your diabetes management. We don't have the space here to discuss every medication on the market, but we can point out some of the more common interactions you'll find.

- Steroids (such as hydrocortisone, prednisone, or dexamethasone) will reduce your sensitivity to insulin and your basal rates, and bolus doses should be changed to reflect this. However, since steroids taken orally won't start acting right away, you'll need to change your basal rates for later in the day. For instance, if you take prednisone in the morning, you'll probably need to raise your basal rates and bolus doses in the afternoon or early evening. If you take prednisone at night, you'll probably have to raise your morning and early afternoon insulin intake. The dosage of the steroid will determine how long the medication will affect your blood glucose levels. Talk with your physician about when and how much you should adjust your basal rates and bolus doses to account for steroids.

- Injected steroids (such as a dose injected into an arthritic joint) are a little harder to predict. Check your blood glucose often and use a correction bolus to cover any high readings.
- Asthma medications such as albuterol (also known as beta adrenergic agonists) and theophylline can also cause your blood glucose to rise.

The menstrual cycle and diabetes

Some women notice that their sensitivity to insulin is different at different points in their menstrual cycle. Usually, in the days right before the menstrual period, sensitivity to insulin will drop and glucose levels will tend to be a little bit higher. Using a higher basal rate during these days will typically help you control this situation.

Women who are on hormone replacement treatment also report differences in their insulin sensitivity during the menstrual cycle. Progesterone, one of the key hormones used in hormone replacement therapy, will reduce your responsiveness to insulin. In most cases, progesterone is only taken on certain days of the month, so basal rates and bolus doses will probably only need to be adjusted on these days. Oral contraceptives can also affect your insulin needs. Talk with your diabetes care team about what you need to do to account for fluctuating glucose levels throughout your menstrual cycle.

Medical conditions

All serious medical conditions (such as pneumonia, heart attacks, and congestive heart failure) prompt your body to release stress hormones, which, as we talked about earlier, causes your body to become less responsive to insulin. If you're suffering from a serious illness, you'll probably need to raise your basal rates and bolus doses.

However, other less acute and more prolonged medical conditions can also have serious impacts on your insulin requirements. Most common are thyroid, kidney, and adrenal disease.

- Thyroid disease is relatively common in people with diabetes. An underactive thyroid usually leads to lower glucose levels, which in turn calls for less insulin. An overactive thyroid causes just the opposite—your glucose levels rise and your need for insulin increases. Symptoms of thyroid disease include unexplained weight gain or loss, fatigue, difficulty handling hot or cold temperatures, nervousness, and constipation. Talk with your diabetes care team if you believe you're suffering from a thyroid condition.

- Kidney failure is unfortunately one of the more common complications of diabetes and can lead to an interesting insulin paradox. On one hand, you'll become less sensitive to insulin and your blood glucose will tend to rise. On the other hand, your body will filter out less insulin, so your overall insulin needs will probably drop. Working closely with your diabetes care team, you will need to determine the best approach to this balancing act.

- Adrenal disease is rare, but not unheard of, especially in people with type 1 diabetes. If you develop adrenal insufficiency, you are prone to hypoglycemia, and your insulin needs will drop. The symptoms of adrenal insufficiency include weight loss, fatigue, and nausea.

11 Nutrition 101:
Food and the Pump

By now you know that of the nutrients you eat, carbohydrate has the biggest impact on your blood glucose and that matching your insulin boluses with the carbohydrates you eat is the cornerstone of your diabetes therapy. We've mentioned some of the basics of carb counting and laid the basic groundwork for working carb counting into your pump therapy. However, as we've also mentioned, not all carbohydrates are the same. Understanding that certain carbs can affect your blood glucose in different ways to others can help you tighten your diabetes control.

Also keep in mind that it's easy for people on the pump to focus so much on carbohydrates, that they lose sight of other nutrition factors that can affect their pump therapy. Just because you're counting carbs doesn't mean you can ignore fat, protein, and other nutrients. Carbohydrate may affect your blood glucose the most dramatically, but it's not the only thing at work in your body.

In this chapter, we'll cover some of the basics of nutrition in general and guide you down the path to a healthy diet. We'll talk about the different types of carbs, how fat and protein can affect your blood glucose levels, the effects of alcohol, and the impact of nutrients and minerals on your diet. Scientists and researchers have come a long way in their understanding of nutrition, and putting this knowledge to work for you can bring important benefits.

Not All Carbs Are Alike— Understanding the Glycemic Index

As you start counting carbs and matching your food boluses with the carb content, you'll find that there are times when what's supposed to happen and what actually happens are quite different. You'll be certain you counted the carbs correctly, calculated your insulin bolus perfectly, and yet still get post-meal glucose levels that are out of your target range. Sometimes, this can be the work of factors outside of your diet, such as the ones we discussed last chapter. Other times it will be the work of different nutrients or alcohol, which we'll get to in just a bit. Or, and many pump users find this surprising, it may actually be the carbohydrate itself. Some carbs are absorbed very rapidly; others take time getting to your bloodstream. Knowing which type of carbohydrate is which may help you determine the approach that will get the best results. Should you bolus before meals or after? Should you use the "extended/square wave" bolus or just a regular bolus? To answer these questions, it helps to know a little bit about another tool—the *glycemic index*.

The glycemic index

The glycemic index is a scientifically based listing of foods that ranks items according to their potential to raise blood glucose levels. While the index is not necessarily required knowledge, having a general idea of how the carbohydrates you eat act in your body can get you a lot closer to tight control.

So how exactly does the index work? Basically, the index compares the general absorption rate of a food to the absorption rate of pure glucose, since pure glucose is just about the fastest acting form of carbohydrate out there. Foods are assigned a number from 1 through 100—the higher the number, the faster it breaks down, and the more quickly the carbohydrate acts. Since pure glucose is the point of comparison, it is assigned the number 100, and all other foods will fall somewhere below this. For instance, a food that has a glycemic index

Glycemic Index Values of Some Sample Foods

In the glycemic index, foods are generally grouped into 3 categories—Low, Medium, and High. Low foods have a value of less than 55, Medium foods fall somewhere between 55 and 70, and High foods have a value greater than 70. Following are some sample foods from each category.

Low		Medium and High	
Apple	38	Watermelon	72
Grapefruit	25	Cantaloupe	65
Pumpernickel bread	51	White bread	70
Converted rice	44	Whole wheat bread	69
Sourdough bread	52	French baguette	95
Oatmeal, old-fashioned	49	Corn Chex cereal	83
Spaghetti	41	Instant cooked rice	87
Skim milk	32	Bagel, plain	72
Whole milk	27	Sucrose (table sugar)	65
Fructose	23	French fries	75

value of 87 will be absorbed much quicker than a food that has a value of 32.

Keep in mind that the glycemic index is a measure of how a carbohydrate acts, not how much carbohydrate you're eating. Just because a food has a low glycemic index doesn't mean that you can just eat as much of it as you want. Whether its glycemic index is 25 or 98, 30 grams of carb should still be treated as 30 grams of carb in your bolus calculations. Also note that a glycemic index value doesn't change with serving size. Fifty grams of apple is going to have the same glycemic index value (38) as 15 grams of apple.

Using the glycemic index to tighten your diabetes control

So what do you do with the glycemic index? Basically, the index is there to let you know how the carbs may act and how you should treat them. Index values probably will not affect the size of your food boluses.

However, they may help you decide *how* to bolus your insulin. If you're eating brown rice, which has a low index, you may need to use the "square wave" or "extended" bolus to spread your insulin out longer.

The index will also help you understand post-meal glucose readings that seem a little out of whack. Let's say you check your glucose levels 2–3 hours after a meal and find that they're higher than you would expect. Looking back, you realize that you had pasta for dinner, which has a low glycemic index value, but didn't use your "square wave" or "extended" bolus. More than likely, the carb from your meal is still making an impact. Or you may find that your glucose spikes very high after eating some Corn Chex cereal or a bagel in the morning. Changing your breakfast to a food with a lower glycemic index (such as oatmeal), which is more slowly absorbed, might be a way to counteract this problem.

Factors that affect the glycemic index

As you look over the glycemic index, you'll probably notice that predicting which foods have a high index value and which have a low index value is no easy task. Foods sometimes referred to as "complex carbohydrates" (such as bread and potatoes) actually break down quickly, while "simple" carbohydrates can take awhile. It may surprise you to learn that the glycemic index of a red-skinned baked potato is 93, while that for orange juice is 46. So the terms "simple" and "complex" can actually be quite misleading and have little bearing on how the food is actually broken down in the body. More important to the glycemic index is the chemical structure of the food. The following factors affect the glycemic index:

- Physical form of the food—thick coatings, such as those on beans and legumes, can act as a barrier to digestive fluids. This results in a lower glycemic index.
- Cooking methods—foods cooked longer will digest quicker, thus al dente pasta will digest slower than very soft pasta.
- Acidity—acids slow down the digestion, which is part of the reason orange juice has such a low glycemic index.
- Fat—fat makes your stomach empty slower. Low-fat versions of food usually have a higher glycemic index.
- Soluble fiber—foods that are high in soluble fiber, such as oatmeal, are digested slower, so their glycemic index value tends to be lower.

- Processing—highly processed foods tend to have a high glycemic index value.
- Pre-meal blood glucose—if your blood glucose is high before you eat, your digestion will be slower and *everything* will be lower on the glycemic index.

So now you should have a basic idea of what the glycemic index is, what affects it, and how you can use it to tighten your control. Remember, the glycemic index is not a substitution for carbohydrate counting. Being able to accurately size up the amount of carbohydrates on your plate is still the key. However, the index is a nice compliment to carb counting and using it properly can help you achieve tight control.

Fat, Protein, Alcohol, Fiber, and Everything In Between

While it may not seem like it as you start pump therapy, there's more to food than just carbohydrates. Granted, carbs have the biggest impact on your blood glucose, but there are a lot of other nutrients you're taking in with carbs—nutrients that can also play a part in your diabetes management. Just because you're counting carbs doesn't mean you can ignore healthy eating. In fact, eating right (and exercising!) can make it much easier to manage your blood glucose.

In the rest of this chapter, we'll talk about all of the other nutrients and dietary variables packed into the food you eat. Some of these nutrients will have a direct effect on how you manage your blood glucose. Others are just an integral part of healthy eating.

Fats

We'll start our journey through the nutrition spectrum with a brief discussion on fats. Over the years, fats have acquired a pretty bad rap. Everywhere you look there's something mentioning the evil and dangers of fats. And to some degree, this negative outlook is deserved. Too much fat in your diet and not enough exercise has been linked to some very nasty conditions, including obesity, heart disease, and high blood pressure (not to mention type 2 diabetes). However, fat is not all bad. In fact, certain fats play a very important role in keeping your body healthy. The key is eating the right kind of fats in the right amount.

So what exactly do fats do? Well, a lot of things. In addition to being a stored source of energy, fats also provide insulation and help transport certain nutrients in your body. Without fats, your body would not be able to properly function. The problem is, most people tend to stock up on fats a little more than they should. Carefully checking the foods you eat for fat content and the type of fat is the cornerstone of a healthy diet.

Fats can also have a big impact on your blood glucose levels. A high-fat meal can dramatically change how glucose is absorbed and taken up by your body and make it difficult to manage blood glucose levels effectively. Keeping an eye out for fat cannot only lead to a healthier diet, it can also make a big difference in your diabetes management.

Where is fat?

In some places, it's obvious. The white blubber running through and around the edges of a steak, a spoonful of butter or margarine, heavy cream, cooking oils; these are all obvious fats, and most people know what they're getting when they include them in their diet. However, some fats are a little less obvious to spot. A lot of people are surprised to find that a regular blueberry muffin is loaded with fat, or that many snack crackers are pretty fatty as well. Fat can be sneaky, but if you're diligent and carefully check the nutrition information on the foods you eat, you can spot where fat is hidden in your diet.

Fats are sneaky in other ways, too. Remember, there's more than one kind of fat to consider; there are 3:

- Monounsaturated
- Polyunsaturated
- Saturated

Knowing which kind you're eating can make a big difference. For example, if you look at the Nutrition Facts on the back of a bottle of olive oil, you'll find that it's pure fat. However, the fat is a *monounsaturated fat*, which is a healthier version of fat. You could eat a slice of red meat with the same amount of fat, but it wouldn't be as healthy because the fats are *saturated fats* (see the box "Fats in Foods" for more). Foods with fat content usually carry all 3 varieties, just in different proportions. Having an understanding of how much good fat you're getting and how much bad fat you're getting is important.

Fats in Foods

▌ **Monounsaturated Fats:** These fats are liquid at room temperature and make up most of the fat in olives and olive oil, canola oil, and nuts. Monounsaturated fats are heart-healthy fats, so if you're going to eat fats, try to stick with monounsaturated.

▌ **Polyunsaturated Fats:** These fats are liquid or soft at room temperature and are found concentrated in mayonnaise, margarine, and corn and soybean oils. These fats aren't quite as healthy as monounsaturated fats, but they're still better for you than saturated fats.

  • *Omega-3 fats*—These fats have received a lot of publicity lately, so there's a good chance you've heard of them. They're a highly polyunsaturated fat found mostly in fatty seafood such as salmon, mackerel, albacore tuna, and bluefish. Because they prevent clotting and sticking within your artery walls, omega-3 fats are a very healthy form of fat.

▌ **Saturated Fats:** These fats are solid at room temperature and are found mostly in animal products, such as red meat, poultry, butter, and whole milk products. They're also found concentrated in coconut, palm, and palm kernel oils, which are often used in processed baked goods. Saturated fats are the least healthy fat because they increase the level of cholesterol in your blood, which increases your risk of heart disease. Try to limit saturated fats in your diet.

  • *Hydrogenated Fats/Trans Fats*—These fats start as liquid fats but are chemically changed to be solid or semi-solid at room temperature, which extends the shelf life of the foods they're in. They're often found concentrated in processed foods such as snack foods, baked goods, margarine, and shortening. As a result, they're very common in today's diets. Since they act like saturated fats, you should also try to limit hydrogenated or trans fats in your diet.

Choose fats wisely!

Fats are essential to a properly functioning body, but only in the right amounts. Too much fat and bad things start to happen. It's recommended that you get no more than 30% or your calories from fat, with less than 10% of that coming from saturated fats. If you normally eat 1,600 calories a day, that equals out to about 53 grams of total fat a day. Talk with your physician and/or a Registered Dietitian to determine how much fat you should be eating every day.

Diabetes and Cardiovascular Disease

Many people with diabetes are surprised to learn that diabetes can increase the risk of heart disease. In fact, heart disease is the number 1 killer of people with diabetes. Making sure your lipid levels (HDL cholesterol, LDL cholesterol, triglycerides) are where they need to be can cut your risk of heart disease dramatically. Talk with your diabetes care team about what you need to do to keep your lipid levels in target ranges.

Also remember that it's not just the amount, but the type of fat, as well. Following are some pointers and helpful hints for working the right kinds of fats in the right amounts into your diet.

- Remember moderation! While we need some fats in our diets, we don't need a lot. They're a concentrated source of calories, and we usually get more than we need.
- Try substituting monounsaturated fats for saturated fats you eat.
- Enjoy fish as a regular part of your diet. Fish is usually lower in fat than red meat and poultry and has the benefit of omega-3 fats.
- Choose low-fat or skim dairy products.
- Choose lean cuts of meat, trim fat you can see, and eat skinless poultry.
- Choose low-fat versions of food products, such as low-fat cheese and ice cream.
- Balance high-fat food choices with low-fat choices later. The "30% rule" applies to the whole diet, not just single foods.
- Use the Nutrition Facts labels on food products to help you make lower-fat choices when you're buying food at the grocery store.
- Go easy on fats you generally add to foods, such as butter and margarine. The fat in these foods can add up quickly. For example, just 1 tablespoon of butter or margarine has about 12 grams of fat and 100 calories. That's a lot of unnecessary fat and calories!

Fat and your pump therapy

During the course of your pump therapy, you may notice that after eating a high-fat meal the night before, your morning blood glucose readings are higher than expected. This is because fat can have a big impact on how your body digests food and reacts to insulin. Fat can affect your glucose in the following 2 ways:

- Fat increases the time it takes for food to empty from your stomach. This means it takes longer for carbohydrate to pass into the intestine, delaying the absorption of glucose into the bloodstream. This slowed absorption not only means you'll get high glucose readings later on, but you may also experience low blood glucose soon after your meal.
- High-fat meals can also cause your body to be less responsive to insulin. This can last for several hours after a meal. The end result is that the 5 units of insulin you bolused for this high-fat meal may not work as well as the 5 units you bolused for a low-fat dinner. In addition, your basal rates may not be as effective, and glucose levels may gradually rise hours after your meal. This is why we suggested in Section II that you eat low-fat meals during basal rate evaluations.

Some practical pointers for handling high-fat meals with the pump

Good record keeping will help a lot. Everybody responds a little bit differently to the foods they eat. Keeping accurate records will help you remember what you tried the last time you ate a particular meal and what your results were.

- It may help to keep a separate little notebook just to jot down notes on your "experiments" with eating different foods.
- Records should include the following:
  - Time of day
  - What type of foods you ate
  - An estimate of carbohydrate grams
  - A note regarding the level of fat
  - Blood glucose levels before and at different times after the meal (2 hours, 4 hours, 6 hours, 8 hours)

It will probably take several experiments with different foods before you get an idea of how you respond to high-fat meals. And make sure you're comfortable with your basal rates. If your basal rates are off, all of this work could be for naught!

Once you get an idea of how you respond to high-fat foods, you'll probably want to start adjusting your bolus doses, and maybe even your basal rates, to compensate for the difference a high-fat meal can make.

Adjusting your bolus for high-fat meals

Start by estimating your food bolus as you normally would with your Insulin-to-Carbohydrate (I:Carb) ratio. With higher-fat meals, it will take longer for your stomach to empty, and the carbohydrate will be absorbed more slowly. You may find that spreading the bolus over time will help compensate for this. If so, keep the following in mind:

- Using a combination of a "normal" and "square wave/extended" bolus or a "dual wave" bolus can be helpful. Talk with your diabetes care team about how to use the "square wave/extended" bolus on your insulin pump.
- You may want to start taking 1/2 of your bolus now and extending the other half of your bolus over the next 2 hours. See how this works, and make adjustments if they're necessary. For example, if you still seem to be "on the low side" a couple hours after eating, but "high" 4–6 hours later, then try taking less of the bolus up front and spreading more of the bolus over time. In addition, you may need a little more insulin than what your I:Carb ratio would calculate.
- If you don't have advanced bolus features on your pump, try dividing your bolus, taking half up front, and taking the other half 2–4 hours later.

Adjusting your basal rate for high-fat meals

Another option you might explore is increasing your basal rate. A lot of people notice that their glucose levels will be high for a relatively long time (sometimes up to 6–8 hours) after eating a high-fat meal. Using the temporary basal rate feature on your pump to increase insulin delivery during this time frame can help with this problem.

- First of all, remember to take a bolus to cover the carbohydrates in the meal.

- Everyone's responses vary, so it's wise to approach changing basal rates carefully. You might want to start by taking an extra 20% over your pre-meal bolus, and spread this out over the 4 hours following your meal. For example, based on your I:Carb ratio, you'll need an 8-unit bolus to cover the carbohydrates in your meal. Since this is a high-fat meal, you'll want to add another 20% (in this case, $0.20 \times 8 = 1.6$): an extra 1.6 units. You'll then want to spread this out over the next 4 hours. This calculates out to an extra 0.4 units/hour for the 4 hours after the meal. So if your usual basal rate is 0.9 units/hour, you would program your pump to give you a temporary basal rate of 1.3 (0.9 + 0.4) units/hour $\times$ 4 hours.
- The key to figuring out how much you need to increase your basal rate and for how long is in carefully watching your glucose levels. If 20% extra didn't seem to do it this time, next time increase it further. Keep in mind though that the extent you need to increase your basal rate will vary with the fat content of the meal. Be especially careful if you're doing this overnight! Until you have a clear sense of how much you need to increase your basal rates, set your alarm clock to check your glucose levels.
- You may find you need to wait 2–4 hours after the meal and *then* start a temporary basal rate increase for 2–4 hours. This makes sense if you've tried setting a basal rate increase at mealtime, only to end up with low blood glucose 2–4 hours after the meal.

Remember, there are *many* things other than the foods you eat that can affect your blood glucose levels. The time of day, exercise, illness, menses, stress—these can all have an impact. And it isn't always the fat in foods that cause unexpected high blood glucose hours after eating. It may be protein (which we'll talk about shortly) or the type of carbohydrates. There are lots of ways your blood glucose can be affected, but there's a good chance you'll find that lots of fat in the food you eat can be a common culprit.

Protein

Protein is another essential nutrient that often gets oversupplied in our bodies. Proteins, in addition to regulating numerous processes in our body, provide the amino acids we need to build and repair tissues. While your body makes some amino acids on its own, others need to come from the food you eat.

Recently, a number of fad diets have professed the wonders of a low-carbohydrate/high-protein diet. These diets promise quick weight loss and increased muscle mass, claiming that this extra protein is the key to this too-good-to-be-true scenario. While we won't discuss the pros and cons of these fad meal plans in this book, we can say that most Americans get more protein than they need without following any specialized diet.

The American Diabetes Association (ADA) currently recommends that people with diabetes get 10–20% of their calories from protein; the U.S. Government's Recommended Dietary Allowance (RDA) is a little bit lower. Generally, the average woman is recommended 50–55 grams a day, while the average man is recommended 60–65 grams. Sounds like a lot, doesn't it? Well, the average American usually eats twice this amount!

So where is all of this protein coming from? Most of the protein people get comes from animal sources and is plentiful in foods like:

- Red meats
- Poultry
- Fish
- Eggs
- Dairy products

However, there are other sources of protein, including:

- Beans
- Peas
- Soy foods
- Nuts
- Seeds

As you can imagine, most of this country's protein intake isn't coming from soy milk; it's coming from meats and animal products. While these sources are good for protein, they're usually bad on your diet, because they're also filled with lots of fat and calories.

A healthy source of protein is skinless chicken or fish. These meats tend to be low in fat, yet high in protein. One ounce of meat contains about 7 grams of protein, so a good 2- to 3-oz piece of fish will get you somewhere between 14–21 grams of protein. Two or 3 of these servings a day will get you the protein you need. Another healthy option is to explore the meatless sources of protein available. Working legumes and soy products into your diet can be an excellent way to get protein without getting a lot of fat and calories to boot. Non-animal sources are also usually high in fiber, which is another bonus. Try and incorporate at least 1 meatless dinner a week into your meal plan.

Protein and blood glucose control

When you digest protein, some of it *is* converted into glucose. However, this process is hard to pin down, and it's difficult to predict just how much protein will turn into glucose. Most of the time, protein shouldn't affect your bolus dose calculations.

However, some people with type 1 have noticed that *large amounts* of protein can raise their glucose levels and in turn their insulin requirements. Usually, this only happens several hours after a meal. More modest protein intake (in keeping with the ADA guidelines) generally will not have a noticeable impact on your glucose levels.

Keep in mind though that protein can have an *indirect* impact on your glucose levels. Protein will trigger your body to release the hormone *glucagon*, and this in turn triggers your liver to release glucose. A physician may have told you, "Include protein in your bedtime snack to avoid hypoglycemia"—this is why.

Alcohol

Okay, we know—alcohol isn't exactly a nutrient. But, it does provide calories and is usually consumed with food, so it makes sense that we discuss it here. Furthermore, alcohol can have a big impact on your blood glucose levels, and you need to be aware of what it can do.

You've probably heard that recent studies have shown alcohol can reduce your risk of heart disease and stroke by as much as 20%. This is true, even for people with diabetes. However, there is one key word you need to remember when it comes to alcohol consumption—*moderation*. Generally, moderate alcohol consumption is defined as no more than 1 drink a day for women and no more than 2 drinks a day for men (see box "What Counts as One Drink?").

What Counts as One Drink?

Moderate alcohol consumption is defined as 1 drink a day for women and 2 drinks a day for men, and is acceptable for most people with diabetes.

One drink of alcohol equals:
- 12 oz of regular beer
- 5 oz of wine
- 1.5 oz of 80-proof distilled spirits

Always check with your physician about alcohol consumption. For some people, drinking alcohol is not advised.

Remember that alcohol can have some very negative consequences when it's consumed in excess. Increased risk for liver, pancreatic, and stomach diseases; high blood pressure; the inability to operate heavy machinery, such as a car—these are all bad side effects of too much alcohol. In addition, alcohol adds empty calories without any good nutrients, and many alcoholic drinks are high in carbs, too. Be sure you know what you'll be getting from your drink before you start tipping the glass.

Alcohol and blood glucose levels

Interestingly, alcohol can have 2 distinctly different effects on your blood glucose levels—it can lead to both hypoglycemia and hyperglycemia. Here's how:

Alcohol can reduce glucose release from the liver, leading to hypoglycemia. When alcohol is being metabolized by the liver (which can happen for hours after a drink), the production of glucose is impaired. This can have a big impact between meals and overnight when your liver is your primary source of glucose. To compensate for this, you should eat a snack to provide glucose for your body. Even 1 drink can impair glucose production in your liver, and this condition can last for hours at a time, so be prepared. Alcohol can also inhibit your recovery from a low blood glucose episode.

Certain alcoholic drinks contain a lot of carbohydrates and can lead to possible hyperglycemia. Drinks mixed with fruit juices or regular sodas can be full of carbs. Beers and sweet wines also contain carbohydrate. Although you would normally use a food bolus to cover the carbs that you eat/drink, alcohol's tendency to cause hypoglycemia makes this a tricky plan. If you're just starting out on pump therapy, it's best not to bolus for this extra carbohydrate.

Carb Content of Some Popular Alcoholic Beverages

Nutrition Facts labels are few and far between on alcoholic beverages. So, it helps to know exactly what you'll be drinking. **Remember!** If you're new to the pump, do not add the extra carb from alcoholic beverages when calculating your bolus dose!

Beverage	Serving Size	Carb Grams	Calories
Ale (5.6% alcohol)	12 oz	17 g	180
Regular beer (5% alcohol)	12 oz	10 g	140
Light beer (4% alcohol)	12 oz	6 g	110
Nonalcoholic beer (less then 0.5% alcohol)	12 oz	15 g	70
Cider, alcoholic (5.5% alcohol)	12 oz	15 g	130
Wine, red (11.5% alcohol)	4 oz	3 g	85
Wine, white (11.5% alcohol)	4 oz	2–4 g	85
Champagne (11.5% alcohol)	4 oz	2 g	85
Wine, nonalcoholic	4 oz	12 g	50
Wine coolers (5% alcohol)	12 oz	30–45 g	200–260
Margarita mix	4 oz	24 g	100
Sherry, dry (18% alcohol)	2 oz	0.5 g	65
Sherry, cream	2 oz	5 g	85
Distilled spirits (bourbon, brandy, gin, rum, scotch, vodka, whiskey)	1.5 oz	0 g	100–125
Coffee liquors	1 oz	10 g	90
Bailey's Irish Cream	1 oz	5 g	95
Crème de Menthe	1 oz	14 g	125
Sambuca	1 oz	7 g	100
Schnapps	1 oz	7 g	100

Guidelines for alcohol and the pump

- Check with your health care provider to see if you have any conditions that would not allow you to drink alcohol.
- Always have food in your stomach when you're drinking alcohol. Food will help slow down the absorption of alcohol into the bloodstream and reduce the amount that reaches your liver at one time.
- As usual, be prepared for hypoglycemia. Make sure you have a carbohydrate snack available in case your blood glucose drops too low.
- As a preventative measure, you may want to set your alarm to wake you a few hours after you go to sleep so you can check your glucose and eat a snack if necessary.
- Monitor, monitor, monitor. Frequent blood glucose checks can prevent a low blood glucose while you're drinking and hours later. Avoid alcohol when you're doing basal rate and bolus evaluations and when your blood glucose is out of control.
- It may be necessary to decrease your overnight basal rate(s) if you drink alcohol in the evening—this will help prevent nighttime hypoglycemia.
- If you've been drinking alcohol, glucagon injections will not be effective for severe hypoglycemic episodes.
- When you are new to pump therapy, **DO NOT** add in the carbohydrate from an alcoholic beverage when calculating your insulin bolus. Remember, alcohol typically causes hypoglycemia. Once you have enough experience to determine how it affects your blood glucose, you'll probably have to take the carbohydrate content of sweetened drinks into consideration. Proceed with caution . . . for example, if your usual I:Carb ratio is 1:10, maybe try using 1:20 if you're bolusing for the carbohydrate mixer in an alcoholic beverage. Always discuss this with your health care provider first.

Fiber

When we first talked about carbohydrates, we listed the different types of carbs you eat. Fiber was one of them. However, fiber is different from other carbohydrates because unlike starch and sugar, fiber *is not* digested and will not turn into glucose after being eaten. So why are we even talk-

> ## Tips for Increasing Fiber in Your Diet
>
> - Choose foods that are whole-grain. Look for the words "whole-grain" in the first ingredient listed on bread and cereal packages. Try to choose at least 1 or 2 whole-grain products each day.
>
> - Choose brown rice over white rice.
>
> - Eat the whole vegetable or fruit. Much of the fiber in these foods is found in the skin. Fruits with edible seeds, like strawberries, also provide a lot of fiber.
>
> - Aim for 2–4 servings of fruit and 3–5 servings of vegetables each day.
>
> - Increase your fiber intake slowly to avoid digestive upset.
>
> - Make sure you drink plenty of water.
>
> - Remember there are many benefits to fiber-rich foods, and some of these are from the other nutrients found in the foods, not just the fiber itself. So work on increasing your fiber by food first rather than relying on supplements!

ing about it? Because fiber is a very important part of a healthy diet and has many benefits.

First of all, a high-fiber diet can greatly reduce your risk for bowel disorders (such as constipation, diverticular disease, and hemorrhoids) and heart disease. Second, foods with fiber add bulk, take longer to chew, and can make you feel full longer, thus making it easier not to overeat. Third, fiber is found only in plant foods, which tend to be low in fat and very nutrient rich. So you can see why eating fiber is an important part of a good diet.

There are 2 main types of fiber—soluble and insoluble—and each has its own specific health benefits. Insoluble fiber is found in whole-grain products, wheat bran, corn bran, and a variety of vegetables and fruits. It adds bulk to your diet and is the kind of fiber that helps your digestion. Soluble fiber is found in oats, dried beans and peas, barley, fruits, and vegetables, and can help lower blood cholesterol levels. However, soluble fiber may also slow the emptying of your stomach and slow your absorption of glucose. When making food choices, don't worry about which fiber is which, just focus on adding a variety of fiber-rich foods.

Vitamins and Minerals

Vitamins and minerals are generally referred to as "micronutrients" because they're only needed in small amounts and don't actually have any calories. As such, they don't provide any energy. However, vitamins and minerals are essential in a good diet because they are a key ingredient to all the processes that take place in your body and work with other nutrients to make everything happen.

Almost all foods contain at least a little of these "micronutrients," but some are noted for being particularly good sources of vitamins and minerals. These foods include vegetables, fruits, whole-grain foods, and low-fat dairy products. Not only are they rich in vitamins and minerals, but they're also low fat and lower in calories. Processed foods like snacks and manufactured baked goods generally tend to be low in "micronutrients" and high in calories and fat.

See the box "Ten Steps Toward a Healthy Diet" for more on packing nutrients into your meal plan.

Ten Steps Toward a Healthy Diet

1. Choose a variety of grains, especially whole-grain foods, each day. Eat 6 or more servings of grain foods each day.

2. Aim for 2–4 servings of fruit each day and 3–5 servings of vegetables each day.

3. Remember variety—different fruit and vegetables are rich in different vitamins and minerals.

4. Eat or drink at least 2–3 servings of low-fat milk or dairy foods each day to get enough calcium intake.

5. Choose moderate portions of lean meat, poultry, fish, dry beans, eggs, and nuts. Two to 3 small servings each day is recommended to ensure adequate intakes of iron and zinc.

6. Replace solid fats, such as butter and margarine, with oils like olive and canola oil.

7. Balance higher-fat foods with lower-fat foods.

8. If you choose to drink alcoholic beverages, do so in moderation—no more than 1 drink per day for women and no more than 2 drinks per day for men.

9. Make sure to drink plenty of water—8–12 cups per day.

10. Increase physical activity! Physical activity and good nutrition work together best to promote a healthy lifestyle. Most recommendations say that adults should get at least 30 minutes of moderate physical activity most or all days of the week.

The Bottom Line

A healthy diet is essential to success with your diabetes and your pump therapy. Knowing what foods can affect your blood glucose levels and how they can affect your blood glucose levels is very important. Not only that, but knowing how to build a healthy diet in general can take you a long way towards your goal of tight diabetes management.

What we've discussed here is only a fraction of the nutrition information out there. For more information on building a healthy diet, and a healthy life, look in the "Resource Section" in the back of the book for supplemental titles that can show you more.

12 Intensive Therapy, Weight Gain, and Getting More Out of Your Exercise

Earlier we mentioned the "myth" that "pump therapy will make you gain weight." To some degree, this myth is both true and false. Pump therapy *can* lead to moderate weight gain. However, pump therapy also makes it much easier to control your weight through diet and exercise.

In this chapter, we'll discuss how intensive therapy can lead to these unwanted pounds and how you can avoid an expanding waistline, as well as more suggestions for pump management with exercise. Just because intensive therapy can make it easier to gain weight doesn't mean that weight gain is inevitable.

Pump Therapy and Weight Gain

Weight gain and intensive insulin therapy in general

Weight gain can be a result of intensive insulin therapy. There are a few reasons for this.

- When your blood glucose rises to about 160–180 mg/dl or above, glucose starts spilling over into your urine, and some of the calories you're taking in are lost without being used for energy. As a result, people with high A1C levels generally tend to eat more calories than their body really needs.

■ Once glucose levels get back into target range (the goal of all intensive therapy), fewer calories are lost. So unless you eat less food or exercise more often, those extra calories you've been eating are going to start adding up. Furthermore, there's evidence that when glucose levels are in target ranges, calories are used more efficiently and you'll need less to provide adequate energy for your body. So now you have the combination of less calories lost and less calories needed working together to pack on a few extra pounds.

■ Adding to this situation is that with tight therapy, you're more prone to hypoglycemia and therefore end up taking in extra calories to raise your blood sugar.

Looks like the cards are stacked against you, doesn't it? Your blood sugar is getting under control, which is great, but you're getting more and more calories and needing even less. Fortunately, this isn't an inevitable fate. Intensive therapy can make it easier to gain weight, but the pump can help you lose extra pounds.

Using the pump to keep off the weight

Pump therapy offers a variety of ways to prevent intensive therapy weight gain:

■ If your pump basal rates are set correctly, there's no need for between-meal snacks. When using long-acting insulin (such as NPH, lente, and ultralente) in injection-based therapy, snacks are often necessary to fend off hypoglycemia between meals; not so with the pump.

■ With pump therapy, you can use exercise more effectively to burn off extra calories (which we'll get to in just a bit), because there's less need for extra snacks to cover the physical activity (snacks that can end up defeating the purpose of exercise!).

■ Since you can more precisely control the amount of insulin you're getting, the pump makes it much easier to go on a diet.

■ This precise control also makes it easier to avoid hypoglycemia, so you don't need as many extra snacks (and calories!) to treat episodes of low blood sugar.

If this is all true, then why do so many people gain weight when they go on the pump?

Many people with diabetes started diabetes management under the "deprivation model"—no sugar, no candy, no soda, no doughnuts, unless you're low and need to raise your blood glucose. With pump therapy, there's a sudden sense of freedom, as if you've been released from diabetes prison and an entire world of food is spread out before you. Unfortunately, this leads a lot of people to think that increased flexibility with food choices means, "I can eat anything I want, whenever I want, in whatever amount I want, and just cover the food with extra insulin!" As you can imagine, this new liberty in dietary choices often leads straight to weight gain.

As you move forward with pump therapy, try not to lose sight of the healthy eating goals all people should strive for—not just people with diabetes. It's easy to get so caught up in carb counting and bolus calculations that you forget there are other things you should be watching for as well, such as fat content and calories. Just because the pump gives you the freedom and ability to eat a box of doughnuts and still keep your glucose under control doesn't mean that you should. Refer back to Chapter 11 for some pointers on healthy eating, and remember—your diet may be as important for your future health as your glucose control.

Let's Get Physical—Exercise and the Pump

So now you can see why you might be turning to exercise shortly after you start pump therapy. The pump allows you to more effectively control your weight with exercise than is possible with injection based therapy.

In Chapter 8, we discussed some of the basic issues you'll encounter when you engage in physical activity with the pump. If you've already used some of the recommendations we made and embarked upon your first exercise session, good for you. You've already made a big first step. However, you probably soon realized that the "basics" weren't going to cover every situation you would have to deal with while exercising. More than likely, you were faced with some blood glucose readings that didn't make any sense and perhaps more questions than answers.

Since every person reacts differently to exercise, and different activities produce different results, we probably won't be able to give you every answer you need. That's for you and your diabetes care team to figure out. But, we can address some of the more advanced exercise issues that people on the pump commonly run into.

As you look to move forward with your therapy and fit more and more exercise into your routine, consider the variables that can affect your blood glucose levels. Stepping back and looking at the many ways your blood glucose can be affected is usually the first step to a solution. Variables that can affect your blood glucose while you exercise include:

- Time of the day
- Your blood glucose when you start exercising
- The timing of your bolus
- Your infusion site location
- The food you've eaten before or during your exercise
- The type, duration, and intensity of your activity
- How fit you are
- How well you're hydrated

Looking at all of these variables, it's no wonder keeping your glucose levels under control can feel confusing and overwhelming. But keep with it. Exercise is good for everybody, especially people with diabetes. Eventually, you'll get the hang of it, just like you did with injection therapy. The key is persistence and patience.

Glucose metabolism and physical activity— a working knowledge

Don't worry, we're not going to discuss in long, boring detail every single chemical reaction that occurs throughout your body during exercise. However, if you have at least a working knowledge of how your body operates, how glucose is metabolized, and how your body turns the fuel you eat into energy you burn, managing your blood glucose (and getting good results at the gym!) can be a little bit easier. The following is a step-by-step explanation of this process:

- The fuel your muscles use for exercise mostly comes from carbohydrates and fat. After being digested from the food you eat, the carbohydrates will be in 2 forms—glucose in your bloodstream (blood glucose) and stored glucose in your muscles and liver (called *glycogen*). The fats being burned will come from fatty acids stored in your fat cells. However, each form of fuel is used at different times in different amounts.

- During the first few minutes of exercise, your muscles use their own stored glycogen as their main source of energy.
- Within the first 5–10 minutes, the liver releases its stored glycogen into the bloodstream, and this becomes the main source of energy for your muscles.
- In people who don't have diabetes, insulin levels drop rapidly once activity starts. This, along with the release of epinephrine (also known as adrenaline), triggers the liver to start releasing glucose into the bloodstream (Fig. 12-1).
- As exercise proceeds, fat becomes the main source of fuel. After 40 minutes, about 35% of the fuel used for exercise is fat; at 4 hours, 70% of the fuel is fat. Once again, the drop in insulin and rising levels of adrenaline trigger the fat to release fatty acids.

FIGURE 12-1   Providing "Fuel" for Physical Activity

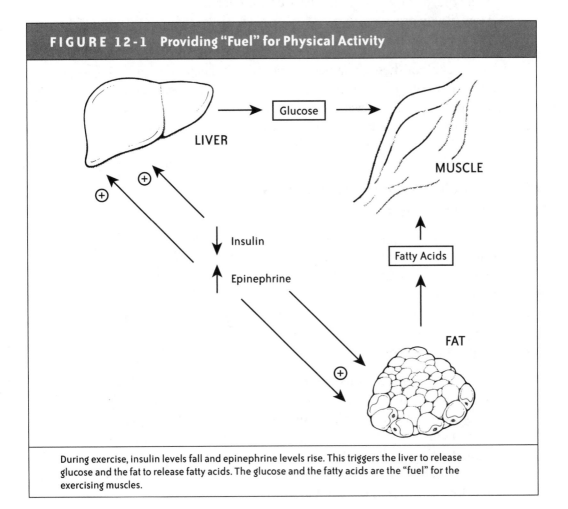

During exercise, insulin levels fall and epinephrine levels rise. This triggers the liver to release glucose and the fat to release fatty acids. The glucose and the fatty acids are the "fuel" for the exercising muscles.

- If insulin levels do not drop with activity, the fat and glucose are not released into the bloodstream and cannot be used as fuel. Instead, the glucose already circulating in the blood is the only source of fuel for exercising muscles, and blood glucose levels drop rapidly.
- After exercise, muscles will continue to take up glucose from the bloodstream to replenish the glycogen stores they used up for activity. In addition, muscles will be more sensitive to insulin.

So what does all of this mean to me?

Basically, during exercise, you're probably going to need less insulin. And after exercise, you'll probably need less insulin and, sometimes, a little snack to keep from going low. In people without diabetes, the pancreas automatically regulates insulin and glucose levels. With the pump, you can do just about the same thing by either setting a temporary basal rate or lowering your bolus dose before exercising, depending on when the activity will take place. Or, you can plan to eat some carb to compensate. It's up to you. Only you know what will work best for you, because only you will know how exercise affects you and your blood glucose levels. Granted, it will take a lot of trial and error, frequent glucose checks, and record keeping, but the results will be well worth it.

Making Sense of Blood Glucose Changes

Change: Decreasing blood glucose during or just after exercise.

Probable cause: Your working muscles are taking up glucose from the bloodstream and are more sensitive to insulin.

Change: Decreasing blood glucose many hours after you exercise.

Probable cause: Your muscles are replenishing the glucose stores used during the exercise and are more sensitive to insulin after exercise.

Change: Increasing blood glucose during exercise.

Probable cause: Your body releases hormones during short, very intense exercise.

Change: Increasing blood glucose with ketones during exercise.

Probable cause: Insulin deficiency.

Some extra help preventing hypoglycemia

Table 12-1 is a sample worksheet you can use to help prevent hypo-glycemia while you exercise. The following example will show you how Steve used the worksheet to help with his exercise routine and how you can use it for your own exercise session.

Steve was training to run a 10K race. He took his training runs before breakfast, around 5 A.M. His pre-run blood glucose usually ran about 150 mg/dl and was usually around 110 mg/dl when he finished his run. These were just the readings he was after. However, Steve was concerned about the time the race would take place—11 A.M. He had never run at this time of the day while on the pump, and he knew that the time of day could have a big impact on how his body responded to exercise. He decided to do an 11 A.M. practice run the weekend before the race to see how he would respond.

The day of the practice run, Steve ate 60 grams of carb for breakfast at 7 A.M., reduced his bolus by 20%, and cut down his basal rate by 60%. At 10:45 A.M., his blood glucose was at 259 mg/dl without ketones, which he figured would be fine.

TABLE 12-1   Physical Activity Worksheet

Blood glucose target AFTER physical activity: _____ mg/dl

Date: _____ Time of day (at 0 min): _____ Type of activity: _____

	Prior to Activity (min)				Start of Activity (min)					After Activity (min)			
	−120	−90	−60	−30	0	30	60	90	120	30	60	90	120
Glucose reading													
Bolus adjustment													
Basal adjustment													
Snack adjustment													
Comments:													

However, at the end of his run, he was shocked to find his blood glucose had dropped to 62 mg/dl! All of a sudden, he wasn't sure if he'd be able to run the race at all. He didn't perform well with the high blood glucose at the beginning of his run, and he definitely did not want to have a low on race day. He called the exercise physiologist at his clinic for help.

Using the advice of the physiologist, Steve did the following:

On race day, he ate 60 grams of carbohydrate for breakfast, just as he did for his practice run. Only this time, he took his *regular* bolus and cut his basal rate by 60%. At 10 A.M., his blood glucose was 166 mg/dl. On the advice of his exercise physiologist, he suspended insulin delivery from his pump at this time. By 10:50 A.M., his blood glucose was 180 mg/dl. During the course of the race, he drank 45 grams of carbohydrate in the form of a sports drink.

At the end of the race, Steve checked his blood glucose and was delighted to find it was 120 mg/dl. Even better, he finished the race almost 4 minutes faster than his goal. Using the information from his run, he filled out his worksheet, shown in Table 12-2.

You don't have to become a competitive athlete to learn how to use pump adjustments to your advantage. By cutting your basal rates appropriately, even a Sunday afternoon walk can be an opportunity to burn off calories.

Some extra help preventing hyperglycemia

While hypoglycemia is the most common worry that comes with exercise, hyperglycemia is also a possibility. There are a few reasons this may happen. The 2 most common are:

- **Insulin deficiency.** This can be a very serious concern if you have type 1 diabetes. As discussed earlier, insulin levels in the blood drop during exercise, and with the pump you can learn to mimic these changes. However, if you reduce your insulin levels too much, or if for some reason your insulin supply is interrupted and you start exercising, the fuel needs of your body will not be met. Remember that dropping insulin levels trigger your body to release fuels into the bloodstream, either through glucose from your liver or fatty acids from your fat cells. However, since your

TABLE 12-2   Steve's Race Day Worksheet

Blood glucose target AFTER physical activity: 101–140 mg/dl

Date: October 15, 2001   Time of day (at 0 min): 11 A.M.   Type of activity: 10K race— Finished in 46:13!

	Prior to Activity (min)				Start of Activity (min)					After Activity (min)			
	-240	**-90**	**-60**	**-30**	**0**	**30**	**60**	**90**	**120**	**0**	**30**	**60**	**90**
Glucose reading	7 A.M. 97		166		180					120			146
Bolus adjustment	1:15 4 u									1:20 4 u			
Basal adjustment	0.5 to 0.2	0.2 u/hr	0 u/hr	0 u/hr	0 u/hr	0 u/hr	0 u/hr			0 u/hr	0 u/hr	0.5 u/hr	
Snack adjustment	Bfst 60 g				45 g sports drink throughout race					Lun 80 g			

Comments: First time to run a race at 11 A.M. since starting the pump. Disconnected for a total of 3 hours. Used a higher I:Carb ratio for lunch. No lows!! Ran well—well-organized race, plenty of water and great people. Overall a success!

insulin levels are low, you will not be able to use these fuels. Making matters worse, when insulin levels are low, your liver will convert the fatty acids in your bloodstream into ketones. Suddenly, you have an extraordinary amount of glucose in your bloodstream, with ketones to boot. As you've probably guessed, the end result of this can be diabetic ketoacidosis. Always be sure you're properly receiving insulin from your pump before you exercise.

■ **Very strenuous exercise.** When you're engaged in intense bursts of very strenuous activity, such as basketball, hockey, weight lifting, or sprinting, your body will respond in the exact opposite way it normally does to exercise. During these strenuous activities, your body will release excessive amounts of *counter-regulatory hormones*, including adrenaline, which do exactly the opposite of insulin and work to increase your blood glucose levels. By both triggering the liver to release stored glucose *and* making your body less sensitive to insulin, they can cause blood glucose levels to rise rapidly. These effects can last for hours. Stress from a competitive activity can also cause your body to release these hormones. For example, a marathon runner might take a little extra insulin on actual race days, as opposed to practice days, to counteract the effects of his race day "jitters" and added stress.

There is another way you can end up with high blood glucose levels after exercising. If you experience a low in the middle of your exercise session and don't realize it, you can have an *exercise rebound*. Just like the rebound effect from common hypoglycemia, an exercise rebound is an increase in glucose levels triggered by a low blood sugar episode. If you have target readings going into your exercise session and end with high

---

Exercise Hyperglycemia

Kim has been using a pump for several years, and has recently begun running. Before this, she had a pretty sedentary lifestyle, and the 3-mile run she was taking was very strenuous exercise for her. She was frustrated that her glucose was always very high after running and met with her exercise physiologist to get some guidance. They agreed on a couple of things:

▮ First, Kim was to check her glucose every mile during exercise to see if her blood glucose had been dropping and then rebounding, resulting in a high post-exercise glucose.

(Continued)

Exercise Hyperglycemia (*Continued*)

▌ Kim didn't detect any lows; instead, she found that her glucose was increasing at every check.

▌ Kim met with her exercise physiologist, and they decided on a new approach. About 20 minutes or so before her run, she began to program a 1- to 2-unit "square wave" bolus, which was delivered over 1 hour. The amount depended on her starting blood glucose.

▌ Kim continued to check her blood glucose before, during, and after running. To her delight, she found much better control with this approach.

▌ As Kim became better trained, and began running longer distances, she realized she needed to change her approach once again. She found she did not need the extra insulin, but instead began to use a temporary basal rate reduction.

Remember, the response to exercise is different from individual to individual; there are no specific rules. Evaluate your own response to exercise and consult your diabetes care team to develop an appropriate plan. As your fitness levels change, you may find that your glucoses respond differently to exercise and you will need a different strategy.

glucose levels, and you're certain your pump is working properly, there's a good chance you suffered a low during your activity and you're experiencing a rebound. Do extra glucose checks during your next session to see if you need more or less insulin.

Rebound Hyperglycemia

Kerry decided to exercise regularly, so she met with her diabetes educator who instructed her on how to use a temporary basal during her exercise sessions. During her first 60-minute session, she used a 30% reduction. Thirty minutes prior to exercise, she decreased the basal from 1.0 to 0.7 units/hour. Her blood glucose was 147 mg/dl before exercise and 258 mg/dl after. She decided she had cut back too much on her basal and next time used a 20% reduction. To her surprise, the results were not much different—133 mg/dl before exercise and 221 mg/dl after exer-

cise. She called her diabetes educator who suspected she was going low during exercise and suggested she monitor every 20 minutes. Kerry was skeptical but agreed to monitor every 20 minutes. She got the following results:

▌ Before exercise—154 mg/dl
▌ 20 minutes into the session—121 mg/dl
▌ 40 minutes into the session—67 mg/dl without any symptoms

This information eventually helped her to determine that she needed to reduce her basal rate by 50% (to 0.5 units/hour) for exercise.

13 Managing Your Pump in the Hospital and On the Road

It would be impossible for us to provide recommendations and advice for pump therapy relating to all of life's unusual situations. Hopefully, the tips, recommendations, and general pump information we've provided throughout the course of this book will give you a good knowledge base from which to work. As situations arise, hopefully what you've learned here, along with the knowledge you gain from working with your diabetes care team, will prepare you for a good deal of day-to-day living with the pump.

However, there are a few situations that sit outside of the realm of day-to-day life, yet are common for people with diabetes. The first is pump management while you're in the hospital and preparing for medical procedures. It's safe to say that for most people, this is not an everyday activity, yet the situation will undoubtedly arise at one time or another, and being prepared can make a big difference in your diabetes management.

The other is traveling with the pump. You'll probably find that traveling and vacations in general can be a lot less stressful with pump therapy. Things like sleeping in and compensating for unusual food and activity levels are much easier to manage with the pump. However, once again, preparation is the key.

Traveling can become a real headache very quickly if you're not adequately prepared.

Managing Your Pump During Hospitalization

Aside from the occasional irritations of dealing with hospital staff who are unfamiliar with the pump and reluctant to let you remain in control of your diabetes, having a pump can make it much easier to manage your diabetes while you're in the hospital.

Remember that inactivity and the stress that comes from surgery or an illness will make you less sensitive to insulin. As a result, your glucose may climb and you may even start to spill ketones. If this is the case, keep the following in mind:

- A few extra correction boluses may be all you need to keep your glucose levels in range. However, your regular Insulin-to-Carbohydrate ratio may not be enough to keep your blood glucose down. If this is the case, use the guidelines in Chapter 9 for bolusing extra insulin.
- If you have a prolonged illness, you may need to increase your basal rate as well. Talk to your physician before making any change to your basal rate.
- If you have type 1 diabetes, remember that you are dependent on an outside source of insulin—without it, you can rapidly develop diabetic ketoacidosis. Even if you can't eat, you *must* continue to have your pump deliver basal insulin.
- Nausea is an early sign of ketoacidosis. If you're feeling nauseated, don't automatically presume that it's related to an illness or that you're coming down with something. Check for ketones. If your glucose levels are higher than normal while you're in the hospital, don't just presume that it's from lack of activity or illness. With all of the moving around that goes on in a hospital, it's not uncommon for pump catheters to become dislodged or kinked.
- If your glucose levels spike while you're in the hospital, be sure to go through your normal troubleshooting routine. And always have extra pump supplies on hand in case there's an emergency.

If you are going to have any type of test or therapy that uses radiation, such as an X-ray or Computed Tomography (CT) scan, be sure to ask the X-ray technician to shield your pump from the radiation.

The pump and surgery

If you plan to undergo any surgery that requires general anesthesia, be sure to check in advance that the anesthesiologist is comfortable with having your insulin pump running during the surgery. Most anesthesiologists are not familiar with insulin pump controls, and some prefer that an alternative form of insulin delivery—such as subcutaneous insulin injections or a continuous insulin IV— be used while you're anesthetized and unable to assist with use of the pump.

Remember that if you have type 1, any interruption in delivery of insulin by your pump could result in diabetic ketoacidosis. *Never* discontinue insulin delivery from your pump until after your insulin IV has been started or you have received a subcutaneous insulin injection.

If you're going to use your pump during surgery or a procedure (such as a colonoscopy), get yourself prepared with this checklist:

- **Reassess your basal rates before the surgery/procedure**. The stress hormones released by your body during the surgery/procedure will make you less sensitive (responsive) to insulin, and generally glucose levels will rise slightly. However, if the basal rates are set too high, your glucose level could end up going low. This isn't something you'd want to happen while you're sedated, so checking your basal rates is always a good idea.
- **Change your catheter the day before the surgery/procedure**. You'll need to be able to check that insulin is infusing properly through the new catheter, so you don't want to put off changing your catheter until just before you go into the hospital.
- **Be sure your catheter is not in a site that will interfere with the surgery/procedure**. For example, with cardiac catheterization procedures, it's important that the pump catheter is well away from the groin and thigh. Check with your physician before the procedure.
- **Apply extra tape to the pump tubing and leave some slack in the tubing**. If the pump should accidentally fall or the tubing is pulled, you don't want the catheter to come out!

Keeping these things in mind can make your hospitalization or surgery go much smoother. In addition, you'll always want to talk with your physician beforehand about any issues concerning the pump and your general diabetes management. Making sure everyone involved is aware of your situation can prevent most problems before they happen.

Traveling with the Pump

Being prepared is the key to ensuring your travels will be healthy and hassle free. More than anything, you need to make sure you have all of the supplies you need, especially if you'll be traveling to an unfamiliar place. In some parts of the world (and even in this country), locating and obtaining pump supplies can be a tricky matter.

Review the following checklist for essential travel items to carry:

- Blood glucose monitoring supplies—meter, strips, lancets, and batteries
- Ketone test strips
- Pump supplies—insulin cartridges/reservoirs, infusion sets, batteries, site preparation supplies, and your pump user's manual. It's always a good idea to pack at least 2–3 times what you think you'll need in terms of pump supplies . . . remember, you cannot purchase these supplies at a store or pharmacy!
- Supplies for going off the pump—syringes, prescription for long-acting insulin, and written insulin dose instructions
- Carbohydrates for low blood glucose and a glucagon emergency kit
- Extra food in case there's unexpected travel delays
- Bottled water to help prevent dehydration while flying
- Documents—letter from your doctor's office detailing your need to wear a pump and carry diabetes care supplies with you (you'll find a sample letter from your physician in Appendix A at the end of the book), prescriptions for insulin, written record of your basal rates, and emergency contact numbers
- Medical identification indicating that you have diabetes

Pack these supplies in a bag that you keep with you at all times. Be sure not to check the bag on airplanes, busses, or trains. Checked bags may be exposed to extreme temperatures and may even be misplaced.

Insulin adjustments while traveling

One of the most confusing aspects of traveling with diabetes is trying to figure out insulin adjustments for time changes. Fortunately, insulin pumps make this a much easier task. Keep in mind that as you travel east or west across time zones, you either gain or lose hours in the day. When you travel east, you lose time, and when you travel west, you gain time. The maximum time difference while traveling across the continental United States will only be 3 hours . . . not such a big deal. For longer trips, however, you will need to give it some consideration. Also, if you have significant changes in your basal rates throughout the day and night, you will need to give time zone changes more thought. See the suggestions below, and talk with your diabetes care team about recommendations before your journey.

When you cross time zones, your pump clock will need to be adjusted:

■ If your basal rates change only slightly over the 24 hours of the day, simply set your pump clock to the time zone of your desti-

---

The Dawn Phenomenon and Time Changes

If you have a pronounced dawn phenomenon, making these pump clock adjustments in stages is important. This is particularly the case when traveling from west to east.

For example, let's say you're traveling from New York to Paris (a 6-hour time difference) and your basal rates are as follows:

▎ Midnight - 3 A.M.: 0.4 units/hour

▎ 3 A.M.–8 A.M.: 0.7 units/hour

▎ 8 A.M.–Midnight: 0.5 units/hour

Let's say instead of adjusting your pump clock in stages (as outlined on the next page), you set the time on the pump clock directly to Paris time when you arrive. That night at midnight Paris time, when your body is still partly on New York time (which is 6 P.M.), your basal rate would decrease to 0.4 units/hour. Now this is close to the 0.5 units/hour your body usually receives around 6 P.M. when you're in New York, so there shouldn't be much of a problem.

However, at 6 A.M. Paris time, your basal rate is now 0.7 units/hour, but your body is still partly on New York time (which is midnight). From midnight until 3 A.M., your body is usually quite insulin sensitive, and you only need 0.4 units/hour. Instead, while you're still sleeping at 6 A.M. in Paris, you're receiving 0.7 units/hour—0.3 units/hour more than you need!

So you can see why it's so important to adjust your pump clock gradually. If you don't, you could end up with a severe reaction while you're asleep and some very out-of-whack glucose levels.

nation sometime during the course of your journey or when you arrive.

- If your basal rates vary dramatically over 24 hours, adjustments can be a little trickier. Instead of setting your pump clock to the time of your destination all at once, it's better to do this in stages (by 1 to 1-1/2 hours every day).

  - Day 1 of your journey—Adjust the pump clock by 1 to 1-1/2 hours (if the time at your place of departure is 8 A.M. and the time at your destination is 11 A.M., set the pump clock to 9:30 A.M.).
  - Day 2 of your journey—Adjust the pump clock by another 1-1/2 hours (this will bring the time on the pump clock to that of your destination).
  - If you'll be traveling across more than 3 time zones, it will take longer to make your adjustments. For example, a 6-hour time change would take 4 days at 1-1/2 hours a day.

Monitor, monitor, monitor!

There's one last thing we need to mention to help ensure your trip is a successful and healthy one. Monitor, monitor, monitor! Plan to check your blood glucose more frequently than usual. This is the only way to really know how the travel, time changes, and change in foods and activity are affecting your blood glucose levels, and it will give you the knowledge to make appropriate decisions regarding your insulin doses.

14 Coming Off the Pump

For one reason or another, there may come a time when you'd like to come off the pump, whether momentarily or for good. Maybe you plan on spending a day at the beach and you don't want to expose your pump to the elements. Maybe you'll be involved in contact sports. Or maybe you've just decided that the pump isn't right for you and your diabetes management; remember, there's no shame in going back to injections. Whatever the reason, there are some important guidelines everyone must follow when coming off the pump, even if it's just for a little while. There are also many issues to consider when you return to the pump. In this chapter, we'll cover some of the basics involved with this starting and stopping and how to make the transition a smooth and safe one.

Taking a Short Break from the Pump

There will probably be times when you'd like to temporarily remove your pump, such as when you play contact sports. During these periods, taking an additional injection of Lantus (glargine) insulin along with the insulin you receive from your pump can be a good way to control your diabetes. The following example should help illustrate how this is done.

Chris is a sophomore at college, a pump user, and an active soccer player. In the past, he'd just remove his pump and take intermittent bolus doses while he was at soccer camp or during games. However, this usually made his glucose levels jump from one extreme to another, which would affect his performance while playing. His basal rates were as follows:

- Midnight–3 A.M.: 0.5 units/hour
- 3 A.M.–8 A.M.: 0.8 units/hour
- 8 A.M.–Midnight: 0.5 units/hour

Chris talked to an exercise physiologist, and under her recommendations, he started taking 5 units of Lantus every evening. To adjust for this extra insulin, Chris determined that on an hour-by-hour basis, this broke down to about 0.2 units/hour (5 units ÷ 24 hours). He then adjusted his basal rate to account for this. His new basal rates were:

- Midnight–3 A.M.: 0.3 units/hour
- 3 A.M.–8 A.M.: 0.6 units/hour
- 8 A.M.–Midnight: 0.3 units/hour

Now, he still has the set-up in his pump basal rates to cover his glucose overnight, but when he takes off his pump for soccer practice and games, he's got the basal insulin provided by the Lantus injections to provide some background insulin. Soon after he made this change, Chris was pleased to find that his glucose levels during soccer were much more stable.

For other pointers on managing your diabetes while taking a short break from the pump, see Chapter 7.

An Extended Vacation

Sometimes, your "break" from the pump can end up being more than a 3-hour breather. On rare occasions, your pump can malfunction, requiring you to return to injection therapy for a few days until you can get a new pump from the manufacturer. Whatever the reason, you have a few therapy options available to you while you're off the pump. You can continue taking your boluses using your Sensitivity Factor (SF) and Insulin-to-Carbohydrate (I:Carb) ratio. However, you'll need extra insulin to cover for your basal rates.

■ If you can get NPH or lente insulin, you can take small injections of this insulin in addition to your boluses at mealtime to provide some basal insulin. You'll need to figure out how much insulin you would regularly be receiving from your pump between meals and then inject this amount with your bolus. For example, let's say your normal basal rate in the morning is 0.5 units per hour. You plan to eat breakfast at 8 A.M. and then lunch at noon. To cover the 4 hours between meals, you'll want to inject 2 units of NPH or lente at breakfast (0.5 units × 4 hours = 2 units) plus your bolus. If you use multiple basal rates, you'll need to calculate how much insulin you'd be receiving for different times of the day. With your dinner, you'll want to take the amount of insulin you'd receive from your basal rate during the period between dinner and bedtime, *not* the amount you'd normally get from dinner until breakfast the next morning. At bedtime, you may want to take more NPH or lente than you would normally receive from your pump, since you generally need more insulin overnight (usually 1.2–1.5 × the amount of basal insulin you'd receive overnight). So if your basal rate would add up to 5.5 units of insulin over the course of the night, you may want to take 6 or 7 units, depending on your own nighttime sensitivity. Talk with your diabetes care team to see what would work best for you.

■ Another alternative is to use a single daily injection of Lantus (glargine) to cover all of your basal needs. If it looks like you're going to be off the pump for awhile, this might be the easiest option. However, because Lantus has an extended action profile, making the transition back to the pump can be more difficult. So if you're only going to be off the pump for a short period, it's best to stick with multiple NPH or lente injections.

If you don't have access to Lantus or NPH/lente, you'll need to get by on the fast-acting insulin you'd normally be receiving from your pump. Once again, you would use your normal I:Carb ratio and SF to determine bolus doses. Basal rates, however, will need to be administered a little differently:

■ If you're using Humalog/Novalog, you would take your pre-meal insulin dose based on your usual I:Carb ratio and SF. In addition, between breakfast and lunch, lunch and supper, and supper and bedtime, you would take an extra injection of Humalog/Novolog that is equal to the amount of basal insulin your pump would give during this time. You also will not be able to take one large injection of insulin at bedtime to cover your nighttime needs. Instead, you'll need to take multiple, small doses every 3–4 hours. Remember to set your alarm and eat plenty of snacks to make sure you don't go low.

■ If you're using regular insulin to cover your needs, you would take your pre-meal dose based on your usual I:Carb ratio and SF. In addition, with each of these pre-meal injections, you would need to take an extra amount of regular, equal to the amount of basal your pump would give you until the next meal. At bedtime, however, you will still not be able to take 1 injection to last through the night. Plan on taking multiple injections at 5- to 6-hour intervals. Once again, remember to set your alarm clock and eat plenty of snacks.

A good way to look at injection therapy while you're off the pump is as a balancing act. On the one hand, you will need insulin in your system *all the time* to ensure that you do not start developing ketones. On the other, you'll need plenty of carbohydrate to make sure you don't develop hypoglycemia. Walking this tightrope can sometimes feel difficult, especially if you've become accustomed to the more "hands-off" approach you can get from the pump. But just because you're taking a break from the pump doesn't mean you should take a break from good diabetes management.

Guidelines for Resuming Pump Therapy

If you decide to come back to the pump, consider the following:

■ Return to your previous pump settings and talk to your pump health care professional. It's best to resume pump therapy in the morning. That way, you have an entire day to troubleshoot if necessary.

■ Check your blood glucose frequently. Closely monitoring your glucose levels will help you detect high and low blood sugars.

■ If you've been taking NPH/lente while off the pump, be sure to take into consideration the blood glucose–lowering effects of the insulin. You may want to *decrease* your NPH/lente injection the night before you start back on pump therapy. Be sure to *elim-*

inate your NPH/lente dose the morning you start back. Talk to a member of your diabetes care team for more.

■ If you've been using long-acting Lantus while off the pump, making the transition back to the pump can be a little trickier than if you'd used NPH/lente. It may be easiest to skip an injection of Lantus the night before you resume pump therapy and take an injection of NPH/lente instead.

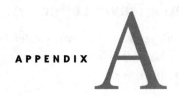

Sample Letters

Sample Travel Letter

Following is a sample travel letter we suggest all pump users carry when traveling. This will help avoid confusions and address any security concerns your pump may raise.

RE: _____

To Whom It May Concern:

_____ has diabetes mellitus managed by an external insulin pump and is under my care.

The insulin pump is a medical necessity for the treatment of his/her diabetes and is worn 24 hours/day. Individuals who use insulin pumps MUST carry the following backup supplies at all times when traveling: insulin syringes, insulin vials or disposable insulin pens, infusion sets, insulin reservoirs with needles attached, injector device, batteries, lancets, blood glucose meter, strips for the meter, and urine ketone strips.

Please feel free to contact me if any further medical information is needed.

Sincerely,

MD's name

MD's phone number

Letter to Your Ophthalmologist

Below is the standard letter we ask patients to have their ophthalmologists complete before starting intensive diabetes therapy with the pump.

Dear Doctor _____:

Your patient, _____, plans to intensify his/her diabetes control with the use of an insulin pump. Studies have demonstrated that good control of diabetes can prevent or delay the chronic complications of diabetes. However, these studies have also shown that tightening blood glucose control can worsen existing diabetic retinopathy. It is recommended that "if retinopathy is at or past the moderate nonproliferative stage…ophthalmologic monitoring before initiation of intensive treatment and at 3-month intervals for 6–12 months thereafter seems appropriate." Also, if "retinopathy is already approaching the high-risk stage, it may be prudent to delay the initiation of intensive treatment until photocoagulation can be completed, particularly if the hemoglobin A1C is high." (**Early Worsening of Diabetic Retinopathy in the Diabetes Control and Complications Trial.** The Diabetes Control and Complications Trial Research Group, *Archives of Ophthalmology* 1998; 116:874–886.)

If you do not see any contraindication to your patient initiating pump therapy based on his/her most recent eye exam, please sign and return.

Sincerely,

Pump Trainer Signature _____

MD Signature _____

B

Insulin Pump and Carb Flowsheets

Insulin Pump and Carb Flowsheet

My insulin:carb ratio:
My sensitivity factor:
I correct a high blood glucose to a target of:

Day/Date	midn	6A	7A	8A	9A	10A	11A	noon	1P	2P	3P	4P	5P	6P	7P	8P	9P	10P	11P
Blood Glucose																			
Basal Rate																			
Carb grams																			
Food bolus																			
Correction bolus																			
Activity: length																			
type																			
Temp basal rate																			
Set change (✓)																			

Notes (pump alarms, how I feel today . . .):

Breakfast and Morning Snack:

Time:	Qty:	Food/Drink:	Carb grams:
			Total Carb:
Time:			
			Total Carb:

Lunch and Afternoon Snack:

Time:	Qty:	Food/Drink:	Carb grams:
			Total Carb:
Time:			
			Total Carb:

Supper and Bedtime Snack:

Time:	Qty:	Food/Drink:	Carb grams:
			Total Carb:
Time:			
			Total Carb:

Insulin Pump Flowsheet for Recording 2 Days

My insulin:carb ratio:
My sensitivity factor:
I correct a high blood glucose to a target of:

Day/Date	midn	6A	7A	8A	9A	10A	11A	noon	1P	2P	3P	4P	5P	6P	7P	8P	9P	10P	11P
Blood Glucose																			
Basal Rate																			
Carb grams																			
Food bolus																			
Correction bolus																			
Activity: length																			
type																			
Temp basal rate																			
Set change (✓)																			

Notes (specific food items, pump alarms, how I feel today . . .):

Day/Date	midn	6A	7A	8A	9A	10A	11A	noon	1P	2P	3P	4P	5P	6P	7P	8P	9P	10P	11P
Blood Glucose																			
Basal Rate																			
Carb grams																			
Food bolus																			
Correction bolus																			
Activity: length																			
type																			
Temp basal rate																			
Set change (✓)																			

Notes (specific food items, pump alarms, how I feel today . . .):

Insulin Pump Flowsheet for Recording 4 Days

Basal Rate(s): _____
_____
_____

My insulin:carb ratio:
My sensitivity factor:
I correct a high blood glucose to a target of:

Day/Date	midn			6A	7A	8A	9A	10A	11A	noon	1P	2P	3P	4P	5P	6P	7P	8P	9P	10P	11P
Blood Glucose																					
Basal Rate																					
Carb grams																					
Food bolus																					
Correction bolus																					
Activity: length																					
type																					
Temp basal rate																					
Set change (✓)																					

Notes (specific food items, exercise, pump alarms, change in basal rates, how I feel today …):

Day/Date	midn			6A	7A	8A	9A	10A	11A	noon	1P	2P	3P	4P	5P	6P	7P	8P	9P	10P	11P
Blood Glucose																					
Basal Rate																					
Carb grams																					
Food bolus																					
Correction bolus																					
Activity: length																					
type																					
Temp basal rate																					
Set change (✓)																					

Notes (specific food items, exercise, pump alarms, change in basal rates, how I feel today …):

Day/Date	midn			6A	7A	8A	9A	10A	11A	noon	1P	2P	3P	4P	5P	6P	7P	8P	9P	10P	11P
Blood Glucose																					
Basal Rate																					
Carb grams																					
Food bolus																					
Correction bolus																					
Activity: length																					
type																					
Temp basal rate																					
Set change (✓)																					

Notes (specific food items, exercise, pump alarms, change in basal rates, how I feel today …):

Day/Date	midn			6A	7A	8A	9A	10A	11A	noon	1P	2P	3P	4P	5P	6P	7P	8P	9P	10P	11P
Blood Glucose																					
Basal Rate																					
Carb grams																					
Food bolus																					
Correction bolus																					
Activity: length																					
type																					
Temp basal rate																					
Set change (✓)																					

Notes (specific food items, exercise, pump alarms, change in basal rates, how I feel today …):

Resource Section

Carb Counting Books

The Diabetes Carbohydrate and Fat Gram Guide. 2nd Edition. Lea Ann Holzmeister, RD, CDE. American Diabetes Association and The American Dietetic Association, 2000.

The American Diabetes Association Guide to Healthy Restaurant Eating. 2nd Edition. Hope S. Warshaw, MMSc, RD, CDE. American Diabetes Association, 2002.

Complete Guide to Convenience Food Counts. Lea Ann Holzmeister, RD, CDE. American Diabetes Association, 2001.

Complete Guide to Carb Counting. Hope S. Warshaw, MMSc, RD, CDE, and Karmeen Kulkarni, MS, RD, CDE. American Diabetes Association, 2001.

More Books by the American Diabetes Association

American Diabetes Association Complete Guide to Diabetes. 2nd Edition. American Diabetes Association, 1999.

Diabetes A to Z. 4th Edition. American Diabetes Association, 2000.

Beating the Blood Sugar Blues: Proven Methods and Wisdom for Controlling Hypoglycemia. Thomas A. Lincoln, MD, and John A. Eaddy, MD. American Diabetes Association, 2001.

101 Tips for Improving Your Blood Sugar. 2nd Edition. University of New Mexico Diabetes Care Team. American Diabetes Association, 1999.

101 Foot Care Tips for People with Diabetes. Jessie H. Ahroni, PhD, ARNP, CDE. American Diabetes Association, 2000.

101 Nutrition Tips for People with Diabetes. Patti B. Geil, MS, RD, FADA, CDE, and Lea Ann Holzmeister, RD, CDE. American Diabetes Association, 1999.

16 Myths of a "Diabetic Diet." Karen Hanson Chalmers, MS, RD, CDE, and Amy E. Peterson, MS, RD, CDE. American Diabetes Association, 1999.

Index

About the American Diabetes Association

The American Diabetes Association is the nation's leading voluntary health organization supporting diabetes research, information, and advocacy. Its mission is to prevent and cure diabetes and to improve the lives of all people affected by diabetes. The American Diabetes Association is the leading publisher of comprehensive diabetes information. Its huge library of practical and authoritative books for people with diabetes covers every aspect of self-care—cooking and nutrition, fitness, weight control, medications, complications, emotional issues, and general self-care.

To order American Diabetes Association books: Call 1-800-232-6733.
http://store.diabetes.org [Note: there is no need to use www when typing this particular Web address]

To join the American Diabetes Association: Call 1-800-806-7801.
www.diabetes.org/membership

For more information about diabetes or ADA programs and services:
Call 1-800-342-2383. E-mail: Customerservice@diabetes.org www.diabetes.org

To locate an ADA/NCQA Recognized Provider of quality diabetes care in your area:
www.ncqa.org/dprp/

To find an ADA Recognized Education Program in your area:
Call 1-888-232-0822. www.diabetes.org/recognition/education.asp

To join the fight to increase funding for diabetes research, end discrimination, and improve insurance coverage: Call 1-800-342-2383. www.diabetes.org/advocacy

To find out how you can get involved with the programs in your community:
Call 1-800-342-2383. See below for program Web addresses.

- American Diabetes Month: Educational activities aimed at those diagnosed with diabetes—month of November. www.diabetes.org/ADM
- American Diabetes Alert: Annual public awareness campaign to find the undiagnosed—held the fourth Tuesday in March. www.diabetes.org/alert
- The Diabetes Assistance & Resources Program (DAR): diabetes awareness program targeted to the Latino community. www.diabetes.org/DAR
- African American Program: diabetes awareness program targeted to the African American community. www.diabetes.org/africanamerican
- Awakening the Spirit: Pathways to Diabetes Prevention & Control: diabetes awareness program targeted to the Native American community. www.diabetes.org/awakening

To find out about an important research project regarding type 2 diabetes:
www.diabetes.org/ada/research.asp

To obtain information on making a planned gift or charitable bequest:
Call 1-888-700-7029. www.diabetes.org/ada/plan.asp

To make a donation or memorial contribution: Call 1-800-342-2383.
www.diabetes.org/ada/cont.asp